DEEP
SLEEP

Complete Rest for Health,

Vitality & Longevity

John R. Harvey, Ph.D.

M. EVANS AND COMPANY, INC.
NEW YORK

*This book is dedicated to the memory of my father, Richard Guille
Harvey Jr., who taught me to work hard, play hard, and sleep well.*

*Richard Guille Harvey Jr.
July 3, 1910 - February 24, 2000*

M. Evans and Company, Inc.
216 East 49th Street, New York, New York 10017

Copyright © 2001 by John R. Harvey. Illustrations copyright © 2001 by Two Pollard Design.
All rights reserved.

Library of Congress Cataloging-in-Publication Data
Harvey, John R.
    Deep sleep : complete rest for health, vitality & longevity / John R.Harvey.
        p. cm.
    Includes index.
    ISBN 0-87131-938-1
    1. Sleep–Health aspects. 2. Sleep disorders. I. Title.
RA786 H325 2001
616.8'498–dc21   2001023419
                                            CIP

Produced by becker&mayer!, Bellevue, Washington
www.beckermayer.com

Edited by Marcie DiPietro
Design and illustrations by Two Pollard Design
Art direction by Kristen Arold
Production management by Cindy Curren
Cover and interior images copyright © 2001 Photodisc Inc.

Manufactured in China

CD recorded by Dennis Scott
Dennis Scott Productions
220 Bramerton Court
Franklin, TN 37069

ACKNOWLEDGEMENTS

If it takes a village to raise a child, it certainly takes a small community to produce a book. Once again I have been blessed with a creative and supportive community that helped with all aspects of this book.

Deborah Baker and Andy Mayer encouraged the development of the original concept of this book. Andy worked his persistent wizardry to secure a publisher. Then Marcie DiPietro, editor at becker&mayer!, stepped in to shepherd and facilitate the long writing process. Her interest, patience, and ever positive and cheerful attitude not only kept the project on track but made it more enjoyable at every step.

My lifelong friend and sleep expert Dr. Merrill Mitler provided a helpful and insightful review of the first four foundation chapters.

Physical therapists Kathy Guzzi and Enid Soto furnished valuable information on the wonderful stretching exercises in Chapter 6. Pastor John Buxton provided a careful and helpful review of Chapter 9 regarding spiritual resources for peaceful sleep. Dennis Scott did his usual masterful production job in blending voice and music on the CD that accompanies this book. The design team at Two Pollard Design has once again created an attractive and soothing cover and interior that fully complement its contents.

I also appreciate the support of my wife, Dawn, who kept our home and family life running smoothly while I was preoccupied with writing. She provided an emotional and physical environment that allowed me to write this book. Now that it is finished, I promise to catch up on all those home improvement projects that have been waiting.

—John Harvey

CONTENTS

---

awake at night,
tired during the day:
a modern epidemic

*A full 45% of adults agree
that they will sleep less in order to accomplish more.*

National Sleep Foundation, 2000 Sleep in America Poll

W hen was the last time you woke up feeling completely rested and refreshed? And when was the last time you felt alert and energetic throughout the day? Do you struggle to climb out of bed in the morning and then battle attacks of fatigue and sleepiness throughout the day? If your answers to these questions are "never," "never," and "always," you are probably not getting enough sleep. And sadly, you have a lot of company. Americans are working more, playing harder, and, unfortunately, sleeping less. Inadequate sleep ruins our physical health, impairs our mental clarity, sabotages our emotional well-being, and diminishes our productivity.

But cutting corners on the time we set aside for sleep is only one problem. Up to 50 percent of the population suffer from insomnia. They toss and turn for what seems to be an eternity before they finally surrender to a fitful sleep. They awaken during the night and can't fall back to sleep. Or they wake up too early in the morning and lie in bed fidgeting and twisting, waiting for an endless night to cease. People suffering from insomnia struggle with fatigue and sleepiness during the day; they dread the onset of night and

Inadequate sleep ruins our physical health, impairs our mental clarity, sabotages our emotional well-being, and diminishes our productivity.

Almost two-thirds of the population report sleep difficulties at least twice a week.

another losing battle for a good night's sleep.

These two problems, sleep deprivation and insomnia, have become a modern epidemic. Almost two-thirds of the population report sleep difficulties at least twice a week. We are accumulating a huge national sleep debt that is injurious to our physical, mental, and emotional health and has a direct negative impact on our economy.

Perhaps more importantly though, we are missing out on the natural energy that follows satisfying sleep. We are lacking the simple feelings of well-being, contentment, and optimism that come after a good night's sleep. We are denying ourselves the health, vitality, and longevity that great sleep can provide. Fortunately, because sleep is a natural process, we can change our behaviors and relearn how to get great sleep. But before we do that, we need to understand the problems of sleep deprivation and insomnia.

THE PROBLEM OF SLEEP DEPRIVATION

The average American gets just under seven hours of sleep, and the trend is quickly moving toward even less. Almost one-third of Americans sleep six and a half hours or less.

There are probably many reasons for this. Electric lights keep us awake. We are literally surrounded by light twenty-four hours a day. This tends to stimulate our brains into wakefulness. Our inner clocks miss the normalizing influence of darkness that for centuries has reset them every day and guided us toward sleep every night.

But in addition to electric light, we also have television, radio, and computers to excite our consciousness at night and to override our natural tendency to sleep. We might stay up watching a movie or go online to check our email one last time. Before we know it we are up way past our bedtime. And when we lie down and try to fall asleep, we find that our mind is filled with so many thoughts that we just can't shut it off. More than 40 percent of Americans admit that they stay up later than they should.

People are working longer days and more night hours. We stay up late to finish our work and get up earlier to go to work. Factories run three shifts a day. Retail stores are open all night long. Catalog stores and Internet retailers offer twenty-four-hour-a-day service. In most businesses there is more and more pressure to provide later hours for customer convenience. The night has become the new frontier of our economy. As we work later and buy and sell through the night, productivity and profitability soar. There are real monetary incentives for working through the night.

There is also a cultural ideal telling us that the more we do, the better it is. We want to work hard, play hard, learn a lot, and be creative. To do all this, we just need enough time, and it seems easy enough to take that time from sleep.

When we lie down and try to fall asleep, we find that our mind is filled with so many thoughts that we just can't shut it off.

There is even a subtle belief that the ability to override sleep is somehow a sign of power or strength.

There are many compelling reasons to steal time from sleep. It's easy to do. We just set an extra-loud alarm. We tell ourselves that we can catch up on our sleep over the weekend. We drink an extra cup of coffee, tea, or soda to lift us through the tired times of the day. If we cut back on our sleep, nothing that dramatic or bad seems to happen right away. We keep going. We even become accustomed to feeling a little tired. We accept it as part of life.

But this is an unfortunate delusion. The effects of inadequate sleep are both immediate and cumulative, and are certainly injurious and dangerous. Sleep is just as basic a physiological need as food and water.

When you don't get enough sleep, you accumulate sleep debt—an unmet need for sleep. If you miss an hour of sleep tonight, you have one hour of sleep debt. If you miss two hours of sleep the next night, you have added two more hours to your sleep debt. As this sleep debt accumulates, you become chronically sleep deprived. Soon your body and brain cry out for sleep. But in the midst of a rapid-fire, twenty-four-seven lifestyle, these cries are often unheard.

THE PROBLEM OF INSOMNIA

Insomnia is defined as an inability to obtain adequate sleep.

Insomnia is defined as an inability to obtain adequate sleep.

There are actually three types of insomnia. The first involves difficulty falling asleep and is known as *sleep onset insomnia.* A person with this type of insomnia will need longer than thirty minutes, often much longer, to fall asleep. The second type involves difficulty staying asleep and is known as *sleep maintenance insomnia.* The person will usually fall asleep normally, but will wake up one or more times during the night and have difficulty falling back to sleep. The person afflicted with the third type of insomnia falls asleep normally but wakes up early and just can't get back to sleep.

There are also two broad categories of insomnia. The first category, *transient insomnia,* usually involves difficulty with sleeping that lasts for a few days. Transient insomnia is usually caused by some stressful event in life, such as a job change, breakup of a relationship, or death of a family member. Problems with sleeping are actually a normal response to stress. Most people will return to a normal sleep pattern after a few days or after the stress is resolved.

The second category is *chronic insomnia,* which means that the difficulties with sleep persist. These difficulties are compounded by anxiety about falling asleep. Insomniacs are so tired during the day that their activity level drops, which makes it even harder to sleep at night. As many as 30 to 35 percent of Americans may suffer from chronic insomnia.

The most common causes of insomnia are stress and bad habits. But insomnia can also be caused by an underly-

The most common causes of insomnia are stress and bad habits.

ing medical problem such as allergies, acid reflux, or chronic pain that interferes with sleep. Insomnia can be caused by psychological problems such as depression or anxiety. Or insomnia can be caused by an underlying sleep disorder. Medical and psychological causes of insomnia will be discussed in the next chapter.

People with sleep onset insomnia will often relate they are so wound up that they just can't fall asleep. Their minds are racing as they rethink the events of the day and worry about tomorrow. Their bodies are so wired with muscular tension and their nervous systems so revved up that it is impossible to sleep. They may also be wracked with strong emotions, anger, or sadness.

One of the worst features of insomnia is that it feeds on itself.

Added to this knot of mental, emotional, and physical tension is the impact of bad habits. People with insomnia often don't exercise. They eat late. They drink coffee or tea late into the day or evening. They might have a drink to calm themselves. Late into the night they pore over their work, watch murders and mayhem on TV, surf the Net, or play computer games. They have an erratic schedule for going to bed and getting up. All these habits interfere with natural, normal, healthy sleep.

One of the worst features of insomnia is that it feeds on itself. The person with insomnia quickly develops worries and anxieties about falling asleep. These thoughts and emotions add to the mental and physical tension that block sleep. As time goes on, the insomniac slides into a pattern of restless nights and tired days as he or she is increasingly deprived of the sleep both brain and body crave.

THE EFFECTS OF SLEEP DEPRIVATION

Sleep deprivation, whether it comes from cutting back on sleep or from insomnia, has a dramatic effect on our thinking abilities, motor skills, and mood. Individuals who are sleep deprived have a decreased ability to concentrate, misperceive sensory input, make careless mistakes, process information more slowly, and have impaired decision-making skills. Sleep deprivation causes a decline in eye-hand coordination and slows reflexes and reaction time. And people who are sleep deprived are definitely more irritable, anxious, depressed, and more easily frustrated. Sleep deprivation also weakens the immune system and increases the likelihood of catching a cold or other disease.

Thousands of accidents are due to sleep deprivation. Assembly-line workers are at particular risk when the combination of sleep deprivation and a monotonous job leads to costly and dangerous accidents. Health-care workers who spend long hours on duty and who are called in to deal with emergencies are often sleep deprived and prone to making mistakes that may put their patients at risk.

Sleep deprivation also affects productivity. Sleepy work-

Individuals who are sleep deprived have a decreased ability to concentrate, misperceive sensory input, make careless mistakes, process information more slowly, and have impaired decision-making skills.

ers can't concentrate as well and have more difficulty listening to and communicating with their coworkers. Tired workers show decreased effectiveness and creativity in dealing with work challenges.

But the most dangerous effects of sleep deprivation occur behind the wheel. As the miles zip by, most people will admit to feeling brief episodes of drowsiness and trying to fight them off with chewing gum, loud music, or fresh air. More than 50 percent of Americans admit to feeling drowsy behind the wheel. The problem is that those brief episodes of drowsiness are not an early warning that you might be sleepy—they are the last thing that occurs before you fall asleep. The National Sleep Foundation estimates that every year more than 100,000 accidents and 1,500 fatalities are caused by falling asleep while driving.

THE BENEFITS OF GREAT SLEEP

While it is important to consider the negative effects of sleep deprivation, it may be more important to consider all the benefits that accrue when we satisfy our body's need for sleep. Just as sleep deprivation drags down our mood, clouds the efficiency of our mind, and detracts from our motor skills, sleep satisfaction improves our performance in all these areas. After a night of great sleep, we face the day with a cheerful mood and a clear mind. Our senses are fully

Just as sleep deprivation drags down our mood, clouds the efficiency of our mind, and detracts from our motor skills, sleep satisfaction improves our performance in all these areas.

alert and ready to enjoy all the sensations around us.

Great sleep sustains our physical health. During a good night's sleep, growth hormone is released into our bloodstream. Worn-out muscles and tissues are repaired. Healing takes place throughout the body. Our immune system fights off invaders and is strengthened to deal with the challenges of the next day. Hormonal levels rebalance and blood chemistry is realigned. Sleep is a period of natural renewal that can increase our daily feelings of health and well-being. Sleep is also a key element in sustaining longevity.

Another benefit of complete sleep is enhanced productivity and creativity. When we are fully rested, we can work efficiently and accurately. We can stay focused longer and get more done. When our brain receives the nourishing rest it needs, we have access to a natural source of creativity.

Sleep is one of our greatest natural resources for health and well-being. But it is one we have to learn to manage. Gone are the times when the environment and daily life supported good sleep. Now there are many environmental influences that work to interfere with satisfying sleep.

We need to make a conscious choice and a sustained effort to improve our sleep. If we do, we can enjoy health, productivity, creativity, and longevity. If we don't and we fall into a pattern of sleep deprivation or chronic insomnia, we will see our mood, health, and creativity decline and we will certainly shorten our life span.

Sleep is a period of natural renewal that can increase our daily feelings of health and well-being.

chapter two

the nature of sleep

and

sleep problems

Come, Sleep! O Sleep, the certain knot of peace,
The baiting-place of wit, the balm of woe,
The poor man's wealth, the prisoner's release,
Th' indifferent judge between the high and low.

Philip Sidney, *Astrophel and Stella*, Sonnet 39

S leep is a universal experience shared by people of all classes, all races, and all ages. Sleep has been our daily companion since the moment of our birth. We know intimately what sleep is because we fall asleep every day. Yet at the same time, we know nothing about it because we lose conscious awareness the instant we drift off to sleep.

The ancients thought of sleep as a kind of "mini death," a nightly journey to a dark land of death with a return to the world of living at daylight. As metaphorical explanations of sleep lost credibility, more mechanical perspectives developed. Sleep was seen as a simple shutdown of normal waking consciousness. It was thought that through some change in either blood circulation or body humors, the brain was put into a passive state of sleep. Or it was believed that with the onset of dark and a lack of environmental stimulation, the brain went to sleep. Only recently have we discovered that sleep is a complex and active brain process.

Sleep is a complex and active brain process.

Scientists in the
1950s determined
that there were
distinct stages
of sleep.

THE MODERN SCIENCE OF SLEEP

The modern science of sleep began in the 1950s when scientists began monitoring the electrical activity of the brain during sleep. They observed very distinct patterns of brain waves and determined that there were distinct stages of sleep, each characterized by a unique type of brain wave.

The Stages of Sleep

To better understand this, consider that your normal waking consciousness consists of fairly fast brain waves in the range of eighteen to twenty-two cycles per second (cps), known as *beta waves*. When your brain is firing in this range, you are alert, aware of the sights and sounds around you, and actively thinking. But if you close your eyes and begin to relax, your brain waves will slow down, increase in amplitude, and settle into the *alpha*, or eight to twelve cps range. You are still awake, but your thoughts may drift and travel and you will feel a pleasant state of relaxation.

Sleep begins as the brain waves slow down to three to seven cps, or the *theta* range. This is *Stage 1* of sleep. It is light sleep. You can be easily roused back to an alert state. But as you slip into this beginning stage of sleep, there is a profound change. Your mind is essentially cut off from the outer world as you close the door on wakefulness and step into the realm of sleep.

This first stage of sleep may include fleeting visual images and physical sensations. You will also experience physical changes as your muscles become more relaxed, your heart rate decreases, your breathing slows, and your body temperature drops. If you were falling asleep at night, you would remain in Stage 1 sleep for only five to ten minutes.

Stage 2 sleep is another stage of light sleep that occurs as your body slows down and relaxes more and your brain waves begin to show two unique patterns, known as *sleep spindles* and *K-complexes.* The sleep spindles are short, two- to three-second bursts of rapid-frequency waves, while K-complexes are large waves that arise and disappear. In this stage of sleep you are more detached from your environ- ment. You can still be easily awak- ened, but you will know that you have been asleep. Typically you spend about ten minutes in Stage 2 sleep.

Stage 3 sleep is the beginning of deep sleep. Large, slow brain waves of one to four cps, known as *delta* waves, begin to take over and the theta waves, sleep spindles, and K- complexes begin to fade away. When these are completely gone and the slow delta waves prevail, you are in Stage 4.

Stage 4 is the deepest stage of sleep. During deep sleep, breathing becomes slow and regular, heart rate slows, blood

During deep sleep, breathing becomes slow and regular, heart rate slows, blood pressure drops, and the muscles are very relaxed.

> The immune system works hard during deep sleep, which is why we often notice recovery from an illness after a good night's sleep.

pressure drops, and the muscles are very relaxed. Growth hormone is secreted, which helps children grow and adults to rebuild muscle cells. The immune system works hard during deep sleep, which is why we often notice recovery from an illness after a good night's sleep. On the other hand, if we are deprived of deep sleep, our muscles might feel stiff and sore the next day because they didn't get the opportunity to heal after the day's work. During Stages 3 and 4 sleep, your senses and mind are completely cut off from the outer world. Consequently, if you are awakened from deep sleep you will feel groggy and disoriented.

REM Sleep

After thirty or more minutes in deep sleep, your brain waves will make yet another change and transition back through Stage 3 to Stage 2. Then a whole new sleep stage arrives, one characterized by rapid eye movements underneath closed eyelids, a complete paralysis of the muscles, and a great deal of brain activity. You are now dreaming. Your brain is so active that you generate some alpha and beta waves normally associated with wakefulness. Fantastic images may parade through your mind. Respiration, heart rate, and blood pressure may rise and fall in response to the theme of the dream. Penile erection may occur in males, and females may have clitoral engorgement as part of autonomic nervous system activation. If you are awakened during dreaming, you will become alert rather quickly and you will remember the content of your dreams.

Dreaming is known as *REM*, or *rapid eye movement*, sleep, while all the other stages are labeled *NREM*, or *non-rapid eye movement*, sleep. Dreaming is known to be of vital importance. Animals deprived of REM sleep will die after several months. Yet the exact function of dreaming remains elusive.

After a period of dreaming, your brain and body have journeyed through one complete cycle of sleep that lasted about ninety minutes. Then the pattern repeats itself. You sink back to Stage 2 sleep, then to Stages 3 and 4. But the contour of the cycle changes as the night progresses. During the second sleep cycle you will spend more time in Stage 2, less time in Stages 3 and 4, and more time dreaming in REM sleep. You will go through four to six of these ninety-minute cycles. You may awaken briefly a few times but not remember it. You will most likely shift your position several times during the night. If you wake up naturally, it will be at the end of your last REM phase with the impressions of your last dream lingering in your mind.

SLEEP AND DAILY CYCLES

This complex pattern of sleep stages is linked to a daily cycle of alertness reflected by small changes in body tem-

The complex pattern of sleep stages is linked to a daily cycle of alertness reflected by changes in body temperature.

perature of 1.5 to 2 degrees Fahrenheit. At 4 A.M. your body temperature reaches a low of approximately 96.5 degrees Fahrenheit and you are at your sleepiest. Your temperature then rises slowly as daylight approaches, and continues to rise throughout the morning hours as you feel more and more alert until midafternoon when it dips; this is a time when you may feel drowsy. Then your temperature rises again to a peak of about 99 degrees Fahrenheit between 6 and 8 P.M. before it starts to decline again to its low point.

There are also hormonal changes linked to this daily cycle. As your temperature drops, levels of *melatonin*, a hormone secreted by the pineal gland, rise and contribute to feelings of sleepiness. In the early morning, blood levels of *cortisol*, a stress hormone, increase and help prepare your body for action.

Your Biological Clock

These intricate daily cycles are controlled by a specific area in the center of the brain known as the *suprachiasmatic nuclei (SCN)*. The SCN is a biological clock within the brain that coordinates all the temperature and hormonal rhythms related to sleep. The SCN is stimulated by the optic nerve, which in turn receives information about night and day from the eyes. The natural cycle of daylight and night constantly resets this internal biological clock. This inner clock appears to coordinate both a tendency for sleep

The natural cycle of daylight and night constantly resets our internal biological clock.

and a tendency for wakefulness. The tendency toward sleep is a constant that starts to accumulate from the moment we wake up. During the day when you are alert and doing things, you are accumulating sleep debt. If you miss some of your sleep one night, this debt builds higher and there is even more pressure to sleep the next night.

The brain-driven tendency for wakefulness occurs in two waves. The first wave comes in the morning, peaking at approximately 9 A.M. This relatively light wave of alertness easily overrides the minimal sleep debt that you have accumulated and you feel alert and energetic. When this wave fades in the afternoon, you may notice your increasing sleep debt taking over as you experience a period of midafternoon drowsiness. But in the late afternoon a second strong wave of alertness comes into effect that peaks at about 9 P.M. When this wave fades after 9 P.M., your sleep debt, which has been accumulating for hours now, takes over. You are likely to feel increasingly drowsy, to want to sleep, and to fall asleep easily.

INDIVIDUAL DIFFERENCES IN SLEEP

Larks and Owls

All of the above describes aspects of sleep that are common to everyone. But along with these similarities, there are many individual differences in sleep. One of the

> The tendency toward sleep is a constant that starts to accumulate from the moment we wake up.

important differences is the preference to be either a lark or an owl. The so-called "larks" are morning people who like to get up early. They feel alert and productive in the morning. But by 10 P.M. the larks are usually starting to yawn and are ready for bed. The "owls," or evening people, struggle to get started in the morning, but become more alert as the day proceeds, and really hit their stride in the afternoon and evening. They often like to stay up until midnight or later. The tendency to be an owl or a lark seems to be part of our basic nature.

Light Sleepers vs. Heavy Sleepers

People also differ in terms of how they transition in and out of sleep. Some people drop off to sleep as soon as their head hits the pillow, while others need time to slow their minds and relax their bodies. In the morning, some people wake up quickly and are ready to jump out of bed, while others need to lie in bed and hit the snooze alarm a few times before they are ready to get up. Also, some people sleep heavily and are never disturbed by sounds or light around them, while others sleep lightly and are easily wakened by noise or light. And different people require different amounts of sleep. There are normal, healthy adults who function perfectly well on five to six hours of sleep, while other adults need nine to ten hours. These variations appear to be part of each of our basic constitutions.

Different people require different amounts of sleep.

Acquired Sleep Habits

There are also facets of our sleep personality that are learned. Families tend to promote a distinct culture regarding sleep. In some families, it is customary to have regular times for going to bed. In other families, bedtimes may be flexible, with children left to retire whenever they are tired and parents on a similar varying schedule. And there are many variations between these two extremes.

Families also promote certain values about sleep. In some families, it is considered a wonderful thing to sleep in on the weekend. In other families, rising early and starting the day bright-eyed and energetic is a great virtue. During childhood we acquire certain beliefs and attitudes about sleep that become part of our sleep personalities.

Age

The amount of sleep we get changes throughout our life span. Newborns sleep sixteen to eighteen hours in a random fashion throughout the day. Gradually, a baby's biological clock becomes aligned with the rhythm of day and night. For several years, young children continue to need a nap during the day and ten or more hours of sleep at night. But by adolescence the need for sleep begins to decrease significantly and most young adults settle into a regular routine of eight hours of sleep a night. By middle age this may decrease to seven hours, and by their sixties and seventies

> During childhood we acquire certain beliefs and attitudes about sleep that become part of our sleep personalities.

most people get by with six hours of sleep at night, supplemented by a nap or two during the day.

The nature of sleep changes with age. Children have a large percentage of deep sleep. But the proportion of deep sleep decreases with age, and by their sixties and seventies most people have very little deep sleep. As we age, sleep becomes lighter and punctuated with more awakenings through the night. The sleep clock doesn't seem to be as efficient in later years. We don't sleep as deeply during the night and may feel more tired during the day.

There are other age-related patterns as well. Young children are often early risers. By the teen years a dramatic shift in sleep patterns takes place. Teenagers like to stay up late and to sleep late. But through adulthood there is a tendency to become more and more of an early riser. Many people in their sixties and seventies are up by 6 or 7 A.M.

Overall, there are genetic, learned, and developmental factors that contribute to our sleep personalities. Understanding these individual differences is an important part of learning to manage sleep.

The Resiliency of Sleep

Normally, sleep is a very resilient and self-correcting phenomenon. Like many other important physiological functions, sleep has multiple mechanisms to keep it functioning correctly. This can be seen in the interplay

Sleep is a very resilient and self-correcting phenomenon.

between the sleep drive and the alerting mechanism. Imagine a night when you go to bed with sinus congestion that makes it hard to breathe, as well as a sore back from overdoing yard work. After a long time of tossing, turning, and struggling to get comfortable, you manage to fall asleep. But then a storm moves through and the crashing thunder wakes you. Your dog barks at the thunder, then crawls under your bed whimpering in terror. All the noise wakes your two children and you have to calm them down and put them back to bed. Later an ambulance drives by with its sirens screaming, to wake you up once again.

In spite of these problems, your sleep drive helped you fall asleep originally and fall back asleep after every awakening. When morning comes, your alerting mechanism kicks in and you are able to get up and function. The alerting mechanism overrides your sleepiness and allows you to carry on through the day. You might not feel great, but you will be able to function. And as the day goes on, your sleep debt will accumulate, making it all the more likely that you will fall asleep easily and make up for the sleep you lost.

In this regard, sleep experts describe what is known as *core sleep*. For most people, obtaining about five and a half hours of sleep gives them most of the crucial deep sleep they need. After core sleep, most people are able to function adequately the next day even if they don't feel great.

The sleep center in our brains also seems to be able to

> For most people, obtaining about five and a half hours of sleep gives them most of the crucial deep sleep they need.

Our brain actively manages our sleep and corrects for anything that is missed.

adjust if we miss a certain stage of sleep. If we miss REM sleep one night, we get more the next night. It seems that our brain actively manages our sleep and corrects for anything that is missed.

We even seem to get pretty good sleep when we mistreat our sleep mechanism. We can drink lots of coffee during the day. Somehow we still manage to adjust and fall asleep. If we drink excessive alcohol or eat too much or too late, we still fall asleep. If we stay up late, leave the radio or TV on, or live in a noisy environment, we still fall asleep. It seems that our sleep mechanism is robust enough to overcome natural, manmade, and self-created obstacles.

Sleep is also very flexible. During an emergency such as a natural disaster or a family crisis, we can override our need for sleep and stay up for long periods of time or get by on core sleep. Eventually we need to recover this lost rest or we become exhausted.

SLEEP PROBLEMS

As resilient and flexible as sleep is, there are a number of sleep problems that can occur. The two most common problems are chronic sleep deprivation and insomnia, which were discussed in Chapter 1.

Psychological and Medical Causes of Insomnia

There are some cases of insomnia that may require additional treatment. For example, when someone suffers from clinical depression or anxiety, one of the primary symptoms is disrupted sleep. The sleep problems are a symptom of another underlying problem. In such situations it is important to treat the underlying mental health problem with psychotherapy and possibly medication. Behavioral treatment of the sleep difficulties may be part of the overall treatment. But often as the anxiety or depression is resolved, sleep improves.

Sometimes insomnia can be caused by or related to an underlying medical condition. For example, if you suffer from allergies, the stuffed-up nose and sneezing can make it difficult to fall asleep and stay asleep. If you suffer from any type of digestive tract problem such as reflux, heartburn, or ulcers, the unpleasant symptoms may disrupt your sleep at night.

If you suffer from any type of chronic pain, you will most likely have difficulty sleeping through the night. *Fibromyalgia* is a pain disorder that involves generalized discomfort in the shoulders, neck, and back along with tenderness and pain in specific spots known as *trigger points*. Patients with fibromyalgia also stuggle to fall asleep and stay asleep, and they usually feel tired throughout the day.

Any type of urinary tract infection or incontinence that

When someone suffers from clinical depression or anxiety, one of the primary symptoms is disrupted sleep.

causes you to get up during the night can disrupt your sleep. Asthma, emphysema, and other lung disorders that interfere with breathing can make it difficult to fall asleep and to sleep soundly. Heart disease can cause chest or arm pain during the night that interferes with sleep. If insomnia is caused by any of these medical problems, it is very important to obtain proper medical care before you use the behavioral sleep improvement methods outlined in this book.

SLEEP DISORDERS

When sleep problems persist for more than thirty days in spite of following behavioral recommendations, it is time to consult a sleep specialist.

Sometimes sleep problems are caused by an underlying medical condition known as a *sleep disorder*. Scientists have identified a number of sleep disorders. Each one seems to be caused by some type of breakdown or abnormality in the sleep mechanism. Sleep disorders are best diagnosed by specialists in sleep medicine. When sleep problems persist for more than thirty days in spite of following behavioral recommendations, it is time to consult a sleep specialist.

Delayed Sleep Phase Syndrome (DSPS)

One sleep disorder is called *delayed sleep phase syndrome (DSPS)*. Individuals afflicted with this disorder find they can't fall asleep until 3 or 4 A.M., then sleep normally for seven or eight hours. They are getting normal sleep, but they can't fit into a nine-to-five job. This disorder is caused when the normal circadian rhythm of sleep is out of alignment with the day. The person with DSPS experiences his or her second wave of alerting much later in the evening and is biologically awake when everybody else is going to sleep.

Advanced Sleep Phase Syndrome (ASPS)

A related disorder is called *advanced sleep phase syndrome (ASPS)*. This occurs when the biological clock is set too early, causing the person to fall asleep early in the evening but wake up by 4 A.M. Persons with ASPS will find themselves wide awake, tossing and turning in the predawn hours while everyone else sleeps. Both of these phase problems can be successfully treated with exposure to bright light at an appropriate time of day to reset the biological clock.

Advanced sleep phase syndrome (ASPS) occurs when the biological clock is set too early.

Restless Legs Syndrome (RLS)

Another disruptive sleep disorder is *restless legs syndrome (RLS)*. The primary complaint is unpleasant, creeping, crawling, even painful sensations in the lower legs that occur as soon as the person tries to go to sleep. These unpleasant sensations can only be relieved by stretching, flexing, and moving the legs or by getting up and moving around. All these responses interfere with the process of getting to sleep. This sleep disorder may be experienced by as much 5 percent of the population. The treatment of RLS may involve medication.

Sleep Apnea

Sleep apnea is a serious sleep disorder that involves a transient cessation of breathing during the night. Many individuals with this disorder stop breathing for short periods of time throughout the night. This disorder is recognized by loud snoring and frequent episodes of stopped breathing that conclude with a lifesaving gasp for breath. The pattern can repeat itself hundreds of times through the night, thoroughly disrupting the sleep cycle, putting tremendous strain on the heart, and dramatically increasing the risk of death due to stroke or heart attack. People who suffer sleep apnea are likely to have periods of extreme sleepiness during the day and as a result are at increased risk for motor vehicle and industrial accidents.

Individuals with sleep apnea are frequently overweight and have high blood pressure. Direct causes of apnea include obstruction of the breathing channels due to enlarged tonsils and fat or extra tissue in the throat. There may also be a malfunction in the part of the brain that controls breathing during sleep. Individuals with sleep apnea need specific treatment for this disorder. This treatment may be as dramatic as surgery to enlarge the

Individuals with sleep apnea stop breathing for short periods of time throughout the night.

airway, or the use of a machine that uses air pressure to hold open the air passages in the nose and throat during the night. Other treatment includes weight loss and avoidance of sleeping on the back, as well as behavioral approaches to improve sleep.

Periodic Limb Movement Disorder (PLMD)

Another serious sleep disorder is *periodic limb movement disorder (PLMD)*. During a sleep study, people afflicted with PLMD will display frequent and repetitive movements of the leg. These may be as minor as flexing the toes or extending the foot or as dramatic as kicking the legs. Sometimes movements of the arms occur as well. The constant movements disrupt sleep and lead to daytime sleepiness.

If you constantly feel tired and your sleeping partner identifies repeated limb movements or episodes of apnea, you should seek an evaluation at a sleep center before you utilize the techniques described in this book.

Narcolepsy

Another unusual and very serious sleep disorder that involves daytime sleepiness is *narcolepsy*. In this disorder, disabling attacks of sleep occur during the day. Individuals suffering from this disorder experience frequent but brief episodes of sleep, generally REM sleep, throughout the day that include the muscular paralysis that normally accompa-

Narcoleptics suffer from disabling attacks of sleep during the day.

nies REM sleep. This paralysis may involve temporary weakness in the face and neck or a complete collapse to the floor. Strong positive and negative emotions may trigger this paralysis. Other symptoms include an inability to move for several minutes after an attack, along with vivid and strange dreams. Narcolepsy seems to be caused by a brain abnormality that is most likely inherited. Narcolepsy must be diagnosed in a sleep center and can be treated with medication.

REM Behavior Disorder

REM behavior disorder occurs when there is a subtle defect in the part of the brain that normally causes paralysis during the dreams of REM sleep. Instead of responding to a dream with the typical harmless twitches, the person afflicted with REM behavior disorder may actually act out the content of the dream, and end up walking into walls and doors. Sometimes people who are polite and normally well controlled during the day become aggressive and violent during the night, pushing, hitting, and even choking their bedmate as they act out the content of their dreams. This disorder is more common among men. Once diagnosed in a sleep center, it can be treated with medication.

Sometimes people who are polite and normally well controlled during the day become aggressive and violent during the night because of REM behavior disorder.

There are additional sleep disorders. Some of them are rare, but all of them are disruptive and potentially dangerous. The reader who believes or is told that he or she has symptoms of a serious sleep disorder should be evaluated in a sleep center. It is very important to differentiate between the many serious sleep disorders and the behavioral sleep problems and insomnia that can be successfully treated with the approaches outlined in this book.

sleep self-assessment: analyzing your sleep habits and behaviors

O sleep! O gentle sleep!
Nature's soft nurse, how have I frighted thee,
That thou no more wilt weigh mine eyelids down
And steep my senses in forgetfulness?
William Shakespeare, *Henry IV, Part 2*

J ust as your fingerprints, handwriting, and eye color are personally unique, so are your sleep habits and behaviors. Knowing about your present sleep patterns is the first step toward improving your sleep.

This self-assessment shouldn't be so scientific that you obsess about tiny details of your sleep. Instead, try to achieve a relaxed self-awareness. If you can observe your sleep in an open, nonjudgmental way, you will learn a lot.

The first question to address is whether or not you are suffering from sleep deprivation. If you are, you need to determine why. Is it because you are simply not getting enough sleep? Or do you have difficulty falling asleep or wake up often during the night?

You need to learn about your sleep personality in terms of optimal periods of alertness and energy and natural times for sleeping. You also need to discover how much sleep you really require in order to feel your best.

Your sleep habits and behaviors are personally unique.

ARE YOU SLEEP DEPRIVED?

The classic signs of sleep deprivation are difficulty getting up in the morning and feeling tired throughout the day. If you are sleep deprived, you may have times during the day when you actually doze off for a minute or two. You may lack energy and feel irritable.

But there are several things that can interfere with an accurate perception of your level of sleep deprivation. You can become so accustomed to being sleep deprived that you accept it as a normal state. You may not even be able to remember a time when you were fully rested, and consequently, you have no basis for comparison.

If you are fighting sleepiness during the day, it is likely that you have developed a variety of strategies to combat your fatigue. These might include caffeine breaks morning, noon, and night. You might keep yourself revved up with exciting work challenges or intense recreational activities. You might surround yourself with bright lights and loud music. You might be so enmeshed in a highly stimulating lifestyle that you are out of touch with your need for sleep.

Consequently, the process of uncovering your sleep debt can be difficult. You need to peer through the dust created by your bustling lifestyle, quiet the noise in your system, and determine just how tired you are. Perhaps the best way to do this would be to stay in an isolated cabin in the

> The classic signs of sleep deprivation are difficulty getting up in the morning and feeling tired throughout the day.

woods for two weeks and sleep as much as you wanted. But how many of us can take two weeks off to study our sleep? We need to find a simple way to assess our daytime sleepiness. One useful approach is the Epworth Sleepiness Scale.

EPWORTH SLEEPINESS SCALE

Rate the likelihood of dozing off in the following situations using this scale: 0=would never doze; 1=slight chance of dozing; 2=moderate chance of dozing; 3=high chance of dozing.

Situation	Chance of dozing
1. Sitting reading	_____
2. Watching TV	_____
3. Sitting inactive in a public place such as a theater, meeting, or lecture	_____
4. As a passenger in a car for an hour without a break	_____
5. Lying down to rest in the afternoon	_____

6. Sitting talking to someone   _____

7. Sitting quietly after lunch   _____
   (when you have not had alcohol)

8. In a car while stopped for a few   _____
   minutes in traffic

Total   _____

The guidelines for interpreting your score are as follows: 0-7 normal sleep function, 8-10 mild sleepiness, 11-15 moderate sleepiness, 16-20 severe sleepiness, 21-24 excessive sleepiness.

A little bit of sleep debt is normal.

This scale reminds us that a little bit of sleep debt, i.e., a score between 0 and 7, is normal. But any score above 8 suggests that you have gone beyond this balance and have excessive sleep debt. A score above 8 also means that you are probably not functioning at your best. And given the fact that most of us underestimate our sleepiness or are so accustomed to it as not to notice it, you could probably add two to four points to your score to get a more accurate reading.

THE SLEEP LATENCY TEST

The most accurate measure of actual sleep debt is a sleep

latency test. In this type of test, you lie down with your eyes closed for twenty minutes at specific intervals during the day in a quiet, dark, comfortable room and measure whether or not you fall asleep and how long it takes. Measurements are typically taken at 10 A.M., 12 noon, 2 P.M., 4 P.M., and possibly 6 P.M.

A sleep latency test is very sensitive to sleep debt. If you are tired and have excessive sleep debt, you will most likely fall asleep in the first five minutes. In the absence of external stimulation, your basic biological need for sleep will take over. If you are completely rested, you will lie there alert for twenty minutes.

You can also conduct a homemade version of the sleep latency test as described by Dr. William Dement in his book *The Promise of Sleep*. Stretch out on a couch in a quiet, dark room. Note the time. Then let one hand hang over the edge of the couch and lightly hold a metal spoon over a plate. When you begin to fall asleep, the muscles in your hand will relax just enough so that you drop the spoon. The clattering noise should wake you up, and a quick check of the time should give you an idea of your sleep latency.

Dr. Dement states that even if you can only conduct this test two or three times during the day, you can still get very good information on whether or not you are sleep deprived. If it is twice a day, he recommends 10 A.M. and 1 P.M. If it is three times a day, he recommends 10 A.M.,

In the absence of external stimulation, your basic biological need for sleep will take over.

12:30 P.M., and 3 P.M. Average your scores and use the following guidelines to interpret your score.

1 to 5 minutes	Severely sleep deprived. A sleep disorder such as insomnia, apnea, or narcolepsy may be the cause.
6 to 10 minutes	Moderately sleep deprived. You may feel drowsy during the afternoon or sleepy while driving and not be functioning at your best.
11 to 15 minutes	Mild to minimal sleep debt. You could benefit from a little more or a little better sleep.
16 to 20 minutes	No sleep debt.

THE STATE OF YOUR SLEEP

If you have significant sleep debt, the next step is to figure out the cause. You can start by looking at your current sleep pattern in a systematic way. The following Sleep Self-Awareness Log can help you gather important information about your sleep. You can fill in items 1 through 3 in the morning and items 4 and 5 during the day or before you go to bed at night. Copy this form, and collect this information for about two weeks.

SLEEP SELF-AWARENESS LOG

Date _____ Day of the Week _____
(Complete in the morning when you get up.)

1. **Bedtime**
   a. Time you started bedtime routine   _____
   b. Time you got into bed to sleep   _____
   c. Approximate time you fell asleep   _____
   Time it took to fall asleep   _____

2. **During the night**
   a. Awakenings during the night

   time awakened   amount of time to fall back asleep

   _____

   _____

   _____

   _____

   b. Total number of awakenings   _____

   Total time awake at night   _____

   c. Comments (dreams, noises, kids, pets, etc.)

   _____

   _____

3. In the morning

   a. Time you woke up   _____

      Total hours of sleep   _____

   b. Time you actually got out of bed   _____

   c. Rate how you felt when you woke up:

    1   2   3   4   5

tired, need sleep / groggy, want more sleep / OK / fairly awake / alert, energized

   d. Rate the overall quality of your sleep:

    1   2   3   4   5

    poor   OK   great

(During the day or before you go to bed, fill in the following.)

4. Rate your alertness at the following times during the day using the scale below.

  (1)   Wide awake and active

  (2)   Functioning at a high level, but not at peak

  (3)   Relaxed, not fully alert or responsive

  (4)   A little foggy, not at peak level

  (5)   Losing interest, winding down

  (6)   Sleepy, prefer to be lying down

  (7)   Hard to stay awake

  (8)   Asleep

( ) ( ) ( )   ( )   ( ) ( ) ( ) ( ) ( )   ( )

6 A.M. 8   10   12 NOON 2 P.M. 4   6   8   10   12 A.M.

5. Note occurrence and time of sleep inhibitors and facilitators in the spaces below.
   a. inhibitors: caffeine (C), alcohol (A), computer use (CT), medication (M), television (TV)
   b. facilitators: exercise (E), relaxation (R), naps (N)

( ) ( ) ( )   ( )   ( ) ( ) ( ) ( ) ( )   ( )

6 A.M. 8   10   12 NOON 2 P.M. 4   6   8   10   12 A.M.

USING YOUR SLEEP SELF-AWARENESS LOG

Your Sleep Patterns

Once you have collected the information, you can begin to analyze your current sleep pattern. The first line of the sleep log has you fill in the day of the week. This will allow you to see how consistent your bedtime is or if it changes through the week or during the weekend. Consistency in going to bed and getting up is very helpful for obtaining good sleep.

Question 1 helps you to determine when you start your bedtime routine, if you have one. It also helps you to identify a time point when you are trying to fall asleep and to determine how long it takes you to fall asleep. Remember, anywhere from five to ten minutes is a normal and healthy interval for falling asleep. If it takes more than twenty minutes, you have a problem with sleep onset.

> Anywhere from five to ten minutes is a normal and healthy interval for falling asleep.

Frequent awakenings may be related to a more serious sleep disorder such as sleep apnea or restless legs syndrome.

Question 2 allows you to explore how well you sleep through the night. You can record the number of times you wake up, the time or times when you wake up, and, most importantly, how long it takes to fall back asleep. There is also a space where you can write comments about anything unusual or significant that affects your sleep during the night.

The information collected in response to Question 2 will help you determine if you have sleep maintenance insomnia. You may realize that stress or some physical problem such as pain or heartburn is waking you. Or you may realize that there is some consistent noise or disturbance in your environment that is waking you. These frequent awakenings may be related to a more serious sleep disorder such as sleep apnea or restless legs syndrome.

Question 3 invites you to look at what happens in the morning. Once you note your wake-up time, you can determine about how much sleep you obtained during the night by checking the time you fell asleep and subtracting any time you were awake during the night. As you collect data over a week or more, you can see if the amount of sleep you receive is consistent or variable. If it varies, see if this difference is linked to the days of the week. Remember, most people get somewhere between seven and nine hours of sleep. If you are consistently sleeping less than seven hours, this may be the cause of your daytime sleepiness.

Waking Up

The information collected from Question 3 can also help you assess if your wake-up time is consistent or if it varies. Individuals with a consistent wake-up time are setting the stage for a more regular sleep pattern. A highly variable wake-up time can contribute to sleep difficulties because your body and biological clock are never able to establish a consistent rhythm of sleep and wakefulness.

Also with this item, you will be able to capture some qualitative information about how you feel in the morning. The ideal is to wake up feeling refreshed, alert, and energized. Frequently, your feelings may fall short of this. Recording your impressions will allow you to see how often you feel rested. More importantly, when you do feel alert and energized, you can look back over the earlier questions and discern the cause. Was it a better bedtime routine? An earlier time to bed? Or a night without interruptions? Similarly, if you feel very tired some mornings, you may be able to identify the causes.

A highly variable wake-up time can contribute to sleep difficulties.

Daytime Sleepiness

Question 4 moves you away from what happened during the night and begins to look at how your alertness fluctuates during the day. Using the Stanford Sleepiness Scale, you can rate your sleepiness at the times indicated. And if you have a strong wave of sleepiness at another time, you can note

Most people reach a depth of sleepiness at about 3 A.M.

that as well. The best thing is to do some of these ratings during the day.

When you review ten to fourteen days of ratings, you may be able to determine if you are suffering from excessive daytime sleepiness. You may also discover there are certain troublesome times of the day when you get particularly sleepy.

Your Sleep Personality

You can also use this data to discover more about your unique sleep personality in terms of your natural times of wakefulness and sleepiness. Most people reach a depth of sleepiness at about 3 A.M., then have a wave of alertness that builds through the morning, followed by a dip in the mid-afternoon, and then a second wave of alertness that lasts into the evening before sleepiness comes on late at night.

When you review your data, you can see how your pattern fits with this general description. You can also determine how dramatically your alertness fluctuates during the daily cycle.

You can use this information to determine if you are a so-called "lark" or a "night owl." "Larks" are simply people who have a strong morning surge of alertness. Their biological clock activates their body early. As a result they are ready to get up early and feel energetic in the morning. Larks often have a more dramatic dip in the afternoon and get sleepy earlier in the evening. If you are a "night owl," you may notice that you rate yourself as foggy or sleepy during the morning but you become more alert as the day goes on. You may experience a minimal dip in the afternoon and a strong and long surge of alertness in the evening.

Sleep Facilitators and Inhibitors

Question 5 is designed to help you identify some of the things that can help or harm your sleep. By noting which of these occur and when they occur, you can get some idea of how your current lifestyle and habits are either supporting your sleep or interfering with it.

Under the category of inhibitors are things commonly known to have a negative impact on sleep, such as caffeine intake and alcohol usage. When you consume a beverage with caffeine, just mark a C on the line at the approximate time. You can note whether the beverage is coffee, tea, or soda. In a similar fashion, scribe an A on the line when you consume alcoholic beverages.

The purpose of this is to help you determine what things might disturb your sleep. For most people, one or two cups of coffee or tea per day will not have a negative impact on sleep as long as they are consumed before 4 P.M. But you may find that you are either more or less sensitive in terms of the amount of caffeine you can tolerate.

Television may be another factor that keeps people up.

Your current lifestyle and habits are either supporting your sleep or interfering with it.

You can note the nights when you watch TV and see if you sleep better when you don't watch TV. Extended hours or late hours of computer usage may keep you up. Note your times of computer usage and see if there are any effects.

Mark down when you take medications. You might code them with specific letters if you take several. Note SM for any medication specifically taken for sleep. Notice the effect your medications have on your sleep.

There may be other things you think interfere with your sleep. Figure out a code letter for each of these things, and track them for a while to see if they are in fact detrimental.

You may already be doing some things that are helping your sleep. Most people sleep better when they do some type of exercise. Write an E on the time line to note when you exercise. You can make up your own codes for different kinds of exercise and record the duration of your exercise if you want. If you set aside time for a period of relaxation, you can indicate that on the time line.

If you nap too long or too frequently during the day, you may find it difficult to fall asleep at night.

Naps can both harm or help your sleep. If you nap too long or too frequently during the day, you may find it difficult to fall asleep at night. On the other hand, if you take a brief nap during the day, you might notice increased levels of alertness following the nap. Mark an N on the time line for any naps. Indicate the duration and try to discern what effect naps have on your sleep and alertness.

If you notice something important about your sleep, write it down. Just by paying attention to your sleep, you may see important connections that will help you understand what type of changes you need to make.

Stimulus Control

Stimulus control refers to an automatic response to an environmental cue. If you are a good sleeper, your bedroom and specifically your bed will be strong cues for going to sleep. Unfortunately, for many people the bed has become a cue for activities besides sleep. For example, many people will watch television in bed. Or they will talk on the telephone, pay bills, or catch up on their work. Or a person might have a computer in the bedroom that is on most of the day. As a result of all these activities, the bed becomes a cue for many different activities and a rather weak cue for sleep.

In fact, sometimes the bed can become a cue for not sleeping. People who suffer from insomnia spend way too much time awake in bed, worrying and feeling anxious about falling asleep. The bed becomes a cue for lying awake and worrying and not for sleeping. Take a moment to consider all the other activities you do either in your bedroom or in your bed.

Ideally your bed should only be a place for sleeping and for sex. Later in the book, we will explore methods to re-create a strong link between your bed and sleep.

Sometimes the bed can become a cue for not sleeping.

Most people who are
good sleepers have a
definite bedtime
routine.

Sometimes a predictable and frequently repeated series of behaviors that lead up to going to bed can become a strong cue for sleep. Most people who are good sleepers have a definite bedtime routine. A typical bedtime routine might consist of turning out the lights around your house, washing your face, flossing and brushing your teeth, changing into your pajamas, getting into bed, reading for a few minutes, and then turning off the light and going to sleep.

A chain of behaviors like this that has been repeated hundreds of times creates a momentum. Each step draws you closer to the end result of falling asleep. The effect is even more powerful if your bedtime routine actually has behaviors that help prepare you for sleep, such as doing a few relaxing stretches.

Sometimes people have bedtime routines that interfere with falling asleep. These might include checking your email, going through your work materials one last time, and watching news about crimes and tragedies on TV.

Think about your typical before-bed behavior and consider whether it is helping or hurting your sleep.

HOW MUCH SLEEP DO YOU NEED?

Up until now you have been collecting information on your current sleep pattern. You know something about your sleep personality. But you are missing one crucial piece of information: How much sleep do you really need?

This question requires some experimentation. If you have been using your Sleep Self-Awareness Log for several weeks, you know on average how much sleep you are getting and your usual bedtime. As a first step, try adding an extra thirty minutes of sleep. Usually, since most people have to get up at a certain time in the morning, this will mean going to bed thirty minutes earlier.

After a week, see if you notice that you are waking up more refreshed and are less sleepy and more alert during the day. If you don't feel much difference or only feel a little better, add another thirty minutes and collect data for another week. Keep adding on time until you get to the point where you wake up refreshed and rested and you don't have periods of sleepiness throughout the day.

Following this procedure, you should be able to discover how much sleep you need. This is the amount of sleep that will allow you to pay off your sleep debt every day, get the rest and healing you need during the night, and feel alert and energetic during the day. You will be able to use the techniques presented in the rest of this book to help you get this ideal amount of sleep every night.

The goal is to get to the point where you wake up refreshed and rested and you don't have periods of sleepiness throughout the day.

pills, supplements, and herbs for sleep and alertness

Not poppy, nor mandragora,
Nor all the drowsy syrups of the world,
Shall ever medicine thee to that sweet sleep

William Shakespeare, *Othello*

S ince the beginning of time, humankind has searched for remedies that would promote a deep, restful sleep at night and a fully alert, energized state during the day. These remedies can be divided into two broad categories: the *hypnotics* that help us drift off to sleep, and the *stimulants* that offer the promise of energy and alertness.

The various substances that we take for sleep or alertness actually parallel a chemical battle that normally takes place in the brain. Our brains produce two distinct groups of chemicals that act either to make us feel alert or to make us feel tired. The relative predominance of one group or the other leads to a feeling of being either alert or tired.

An area deep in the brain stem, known as the *reticular activating system (RAS)*, orchestrates this drama. Brain cells from the RAS interact with neurons throughout the brain. The brain cells from the RAS provide the rest of the brain with neurotransmitters that create a general state of arousal. The cells from the RAS are closely connected with the *limbic system* or emotional center of the brain, which is why states of alertness and tiredness are not just physical and

When we feel
alert and energized,
we also feel happy,
enthusiastic, and
motivated.

mechanical but have a distinct feeling or emotional tone to them. In other words, thanks to all these connections the RAS makes, when we feel alert and energized, we also feel happy, enthusiastic, and motivated.

There are four major neurotransmitters involved in this brain activation, each providing a different component to the experience of arousal. *Norepinephrine* provides general physiological arousal. *Dopamine* provides a sense of pleasure and facilitates body movement. *Serotonin* helps to create the positive mood and enthusiasm that go with alertness. *Acetycholine* facilitates muscle movement. When all four of these neurotransmitters are present, as they should be after a good night's sleep, we experience a sense of physical vitality and positive emotional energy.

This chemical excitatory system in the brain is counterbalanced by a braking system. One component of this braking system is *GABA receptors*, which are prevalent throughout the brain. As these GABA receptors become activated, they tend to slow down overall brain responsiveness and decrease the speed of information processing. This results in a less energetic and motivated state. Alcohol and most sleeping medications target GABA receptors.

Another component of the braking system is *adenosine*, a molecule that is left over when the brain consumes energy during hard work. This molecule acts to slow brain activity, and accumulates the longer we are awake and active.

When we sleep, the excitatory chemicals are replenished. When we wake up, these excitatory chemicals energize us physically and emotionally. As the day wears on, the braking mechanism slows our brains down. It is at this time that we may be inclined to look for a stimulant to help us keep our physical and emotional edge.

CAFFEINE AND OTHER STIMULANTS

Caffeine is the most widely used stimulant in the world. Each year, more than 1 billion pounds of tea leaves and 300 million pounds of coffee beans are consumed worldwide. Almost every culture has social rituals connected with the consumption of these beverages, ranging from the American coffee break to English teatime.

The molecular structure of caffeine is similar to that of adenosine. Caffeine molecules flow to the gap between brain cells, taking the place of adenosine and effectively blocking the braking action of adenosine. When this braking action of adenosine is interrupted, levels of norepinephrine and dopamine rise, providing a feeling of heightened energy and emotional pleasure.

Caffeine moves quickly into the brain, taking effect within fifteen minutes of consumption. It increases overall brain activity, heart rate and blood pressure, respiratory rate, production of stomach acid, and urinary output. In a more general sense, caffeine increases alertness and enhances the ability to sustain attention. Subjectively, caffeine creates a positive emotional state of energy and enthusiasm.

There are at least four ways of using caffeine. The first is to drink a caffeinated beverage first thing in the morning. This has the effect of piggybacking on and strengthening our natural morning surge of alertness and overriding any lingering sleep debt. Another favorite use of caffeine is to counteract the natural midafternoon dip in alertness. Another use for caffeine is to keep us going late at night. Finally, there are some people who drink coffee continuously throughout the day to maintain a constant high level of motivation and activity.

The effects of caffeine persist for three to six hours, and it may be twelve to twenty-four hours before it is completely cleared from the body. Caffeine can produce side effects including a jittery feeling, frequent urination, and stomach irritation. Caffeine also creates a mild physical addiction, and regular consumers who try to stop will notice the onset of headaches, irritability, and fatigue. Caffeine affects sleep by increasing the time needed to fall asleep, decreasing the amount of time in slow-wave sleep, and increasing restlessness during the night. The effects of caffeine vary from person to person, with some individuals being very sensitive and others able to tolerate large doses. People also can become habituated to caffeine and thus need

Caffeine affects sleep by increasing the time needed to fall asleep and by increasing restlessness during the night.

stronger doses to achieve the same effect.

You can avoid these negative consequences and enjoy the positive benefits of a mild lift with judicious consumption of caffeinated beverages. If you have good sleep habits and are well rested, a caffeinated beverage can be a refreshing boost. If, on the other hand, you regularly do not get good sleep and you begin to rely on caffeine to enhance your alertness, you are likely to consume too much caffeine, to further disrupt your sleep, and to develop both psychological and physiological dependence.

Most people can tolerate up to 250 milligrams of caffeine a day. If you consume the caffeine early in the day, you may get an energizing lift with no ill effect on your sleep. If you consume between 250 and 500 milligrams per day, it will have a negative effect on sleep and you need to cut back. If you consume over 500 milligrams a day, you are definitely interfering with the length and quality of your sleep and you must cut back.

A typical eight-ounce cup of gourmet or *arabica* coffee has 80 to 120 milligrams of caffeine, depending on the type of bean and the manner of roasting. A cup of coffee made from the more common *robusta* bean may have 100 to 240 milligrams of caffeine. A cup of tea can contain 40 to 90 milligrams. Many sodas have doses of caffeine ranging from 30 to 60 milligrams per twelve-ounce serving. Many pain medications contain caffeine. An eight-ounce chocolate bar

If you have good sleep habits and are well rested, a caffeinated beverage can be a refreshing boost.

has the equivalent of about 30 milligrams of caffeine.

Monitor your caffeine intake for several days. Notice how much you are ingesting from coffee, tea, sodas, candy, and medicine. If the total is over 250 milligrams, you may want to start a systematic approach to reducing caffeine.

The first change is to eliminate caffeine after 4 P.M. Then cut back on the total amount of caffeine. Substitute beverages that are lower in caffeine by drinking tea instead of coffee, or milder coffee. Then you can begin to substitute noncaffeinated beverages such as water, juice, or even decaffeinated coffee. If you feel tired, you can do a few exercises to give yourself an energy boost. If you have any serious difficulties with your sleep, you should eliminate caffeine completely.

If you have any serious difficulties with your sleep, you should eliminate caffeine completely.

Nicotine

Nicotine, a key ingredient in tobacco, is a potent stimulant. It raises levels of brain chemicals that cause an immediate increase in heart rate and blood pressure. Nicotine enhances alertness and decreases sleepiness.

Unfortunately, nicotine is physically addictive. The most common delivery system for nicotine, tobacco, is harmful to your health in many ways. Furthermore, nicotine can have a negative impact on sleep. Individuals who smoke a pack of cigarettes a day will need more time to fall asleep and have less

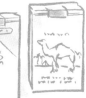

deep sleep, less oxygen absorption, and more congestion and snoring. Anyone who is concerned about his or her sleep should quit smoking.

Amphetamines

Amphetamines, often referred to as "speed," act by stimulating nerve cells to increase production of dopamine and norepinephrine. The result is abundant energy, euphoria, improved concentration and alertness, enhanced sensory experience, and decreased hunger. Physical effects include increased heart rate and higher blood pressure.

People use amphetamines to study all night, to stay awake while driving, and to lose weight. Amphetamines produce tolerance so more and more is needed to create the same effect. High doses can lead to paranoia, psychosis, stroke, or heart attack.

As attractive as the idea of a stimulant may be, the reality is that all stimulants have side effects and either create or add to sleep problems. If we want real vitality and energy without side effects, the best option is to get a good night's sleep.

HYPNOTICS

Through the ages, humans have searched for a substance to overcome the acute misery of sleeplessness. The ancient

All stimulants have side effects and either create or add to sleep problems.

Greeks and Romans used alcohol, opium, and morphine to help with sleep onset. During the Victorian era, laudanum, a tincture of opium, was a popular sleep aid. But it was addictive and had harmful side effects. Other popular sleep aids of the era peddled by patent medicine salesmen primarily consisted of alcohol.

Alcohol

Alcohol continues to be used as a sleep aid. Many people believe that a "night cap" can help them relax and drift off to sleep. Alcohol is a central nervous system depressant and a drink or two can make a person feel mellow and drowsy and might help with sleep onset. But alcohol tends to decrease REM sleep and later in the night it may lead to restlessness, wakefulness, and a need to urinate. Alcohol may also increase snoring by relaxing the throat muscles.

The effects of alcohol are also quite variable from person to person. The impact of alcohol tends to increase with the amount of sleep debt a person is carrying. People who begin to depend on a drink to help them fall asleep are becoming both physically and psychologically dependent.

Sleeping Pills

The first modern sleeping medicine was *chloral hydrate*, a

Alcohol may lead to restlessness, wakefulness, and a need to urinate.

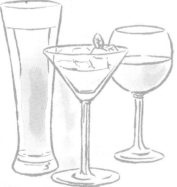

strong CNS depressant developed in 1869. But it was so strong that it was often used as a knockout drug to shanghai sailors. With regular use it was addictive, and an overdose could be lethal.

In the early 1900s *barbiturates* were developed and used as sleeping medicine. Chemically, this medication would affect GABA receptors to cause a broad depression of nerve activity. Barbiturates also created a high, lowered inhibitions, and were significantly addictive. Users would quickly habituate and require higher doses. But at high doses, barbiturates could lead to a fatal depression of the CNS. The common trade names of barbiturates are Seconal, Amytal, and Nembutal. Barbiturates were prescribed up to the 1970s and probably were the medicine that gave sleeping pills a bad reputation.

At high doses, barbiturates could lead to a fatal depression of the CNS.

Benzodiazepines

The next advance in sleeping pills came with a family of drugs known as *benzodiazepines* (BZs). These drugs were actually designed and approved by the FDA to reduce anxiety. Two of the most common antianxiety drugs in this family are Valium and Xanax. These drugs reduce anxiety by a more selective action on the GABA receptors, slowing down the brain waves, reducing worries, and relaxing the muscles. These effects also help individuals drift off to sleep, increase the total amount of sleep, and decrease the number

PILLS, SUPPLEMENTS, AND HERBS

BZs have a harmful effect on sleep architecture by decreasing the amount of deep sleep

and frequency of nighttime awakenings. BZs that are used specifically as sleeping pills include Halcion, Restoril, and Dalmane.

But BZs have a number of drawbacks. First of all, they are only moderately effective. They also have a harmful effect on sleep architecture by decreasing the amount of deep sleep and increasing the amount of Stage 2 sleep. Many BZs stay in the bloodstream for twelve or more hours and can create a drug hangover the next day, with decreased coordination, less alertness, and impaired memory. This drug hangover is more pronounced in the elderly. BZs can also create a range of uncomfortable side effects, including dizziness, nausea, and blurred vision.

BZs can lead to tolerance. After four to six weeks the brain becomes used to the effects and larger doses are needed. BZs lead to physical dependence and can create psychological dependence. Finally, a person who stops taking them may experience what is known as *rebound insomnia* or more difficulty falling asleep. Given these negative effects, BZs should only be used on a short-term basis.

A new class of sleeping pills, the *imidazopryidines* are similar to BZs but have an even more selective effect on the GABA receptors. Ambien, the first member of this family, is being widely used because it is effective, has few side effects, and doesn't harm sleep architecture. Ambien is short-acting, out of the bloodstream in three to five hours, and doesn't cause a hangover. But extended use of Ambien can still lead to physical and psychological dependence. Future medications in this family may be even better.

Antidepressants

Another approach is the use of a type of antidepressants known as *tricyclics*. In low doses these medications have a sedating effect and help people fall asleep and stay asleep longer. Common names for these medications include Elavil, Desyrel, and Anafranil. Tricyclics don't harm sleep architecture, don't lead to physical dependency, and don't cause rebound insomnia. However, they do produce other side effects including a dry mouth, constipation, urinary frequency, blurred vision, and heart irregularities. Sometimes the beneficial effects wear off quickly.

Over-the-Counter Medications

Over-the-counter (OTC) sleep medications such as Sominex, Nytol, and Unisom are composed mainly of *antihistamines*, a medication originally designed to combat allergies that also causes drowsiness. Most authorities in the field of sleep agree that there is no consistent proof that antihistamines really help with sleep onset or duration. They remain in the bloodstream for a long time and can readily cause daytime sedation. They also have a number of harmful side effects, including dizziness, dry mouth, gastric

There is no consistent proof that antihistamines really help with sleep onset or duration.

distress, decreased REM sleep, and rebound insomnia.

Newer OTC sleep medications such as Tylenol PM and Anacin PM combine a pain-reducing medication with an antihistamine. These medications are designed to eliminate any headaches or body pain that might interfere with sleep as well as to provide the sedating effect of an antihistamine. If pain is indeed an obstacle to sleep, these medications may provide some help. But pain may be just as effectively reduced with several tablets of aspirin.

The Pros and Cons of Using Sleeping Pills

Some of the earlier sleeping medications such as the barbiturates gave sleeping pills a bad name. Many people came to associate taking sleeping pills with physical addiction and psychological dependency. But modern sleeping pills, including the short-acting BZs, Ambien, and antidepressants, are relatively safe and can definitely help with sleep onset and sleep duration. There are a number of situations where short-term use of these medications can be very beneficial and entirely appropriate.

One situation would be in the case of a stressful event such as the loss of a loved one. A sleeping pill would help you get a decent night's sleep so you could get up the next day able to cope.

Sleep medication can also play an important part in a comprehensive program to conquer insomnia. Sometimes

Modern sleeping pills are relatively safe and can definitely help with sleep onset and sleep duration.

the worst part of insomnia is dreading another sleepless night, fearing you won't be able to fall asleep and believing that you can't do anything to help yourself. Medication can help you break this cycle and fall asleep.

Over the long haul, medication can never provide the benefits of a lifestyle that supports natural, healthy sleep.

With an effective sleeping pill, you know you will fall asleep. This will ease your fears, break the negative conditioning, help realign your biological clock, and give you time so the behavioral interventions can begin to work. Once you have reestablished a regular and restful sleep pattern and have formed healthy habits to support natural sleep, you can cut back and then eliminate the medication.

Ultimately, sleeping pills should be seen as one tool in a comprehensive approach to managing sleep. They can be an effective short-term intervention. In the right situation, they should be used without guilt or apprehension. But over the long haul, medication can never provide the benefits of a lifestyle that supports natural, healthy sleep.

NATURAL HYPNOTICS

Melatonin

The most recent "natural" sleeping pill to attract attention is melatonin, a natural hormone secreted from the pineal gland in the brain. In healthy people with a normal sleep pattern, melatonin levels are lowest during the daytime, increase during the evening, and reach a peak during sleep.

Melatonin seems to prepare the body for sleep by decreasing body temperature, lowering metabolism, and initiating drowsiness.

Some people insist that taking a melatonin supplement in the evening helps with sleep onset and maintenance. Along the same lines, melatonin has been touted as a remedy for jet lag after intercontinental travel.

Unfortunately, the effects of melatonin have not been thoroughly and conclusively studied. There are no guidelines regarding dosage or timing. There may be side effects with melatonin including headaches, nausea, and giddiness. Melatonin also constricts coronary arteries, which may create problems for individuals with hypertension or heart disease. All of its actions are not known. It may affect the human reproductive system in that it causes regression of the testes and ovaries. At this point, not enough is known about melatonin to use it as a sleeping pill.

Not enough is known about melatonin to use it as a sleeping pill.

Herbs

There are also several herbs that are reputed to help with sleep. Chamomile is thought to be a natural sedative. Valerian root eases tension and anxiety and is reputed to help with sleep onset. Kava kava is a traditional Polynesian remedy that is known to reduce anxiety and create relaxation. It may also help with sleep onset.

One challenge that exists in using these herbs is determining the right dosage and timing. Consequently, if you are interested in using herbs to help with your sleep, you may want to consult with a physician or health practitioner knowledgeable and experienced with herbs and natural remedies.

the first step:
managing time and
creating an optimal
sleep environment

Stick to a regular schedule of going to bed
and getting up at the same time every day.

Elizabeth and Merrill Mitler, *101 Questions about Sleep & Dreams*

T he first step in improving your sleep is to create the most favorable sleep environment possible, to align your sleep with your biological clock, and to establish a regular sleep schedule. Many sleep problems are due to a disruptive sleep environment and to poor habits regarding time. Changing these counterproductive habits will quickly lead to improvements in your sleep.

But these changes should be done gently. Sleep is meant to be an enjoyment in life. Move easily and comfortably but actively and persistently to improve your sleep.

CREATING AN OPTIMAL SLEEP ENVIRONMENT

Considering that you spend anywhere from one-quarter to one-third of your life sleeping, it makes good sense to design your bedroom to promote great sleep. All too often a bedroom has many uses. Some people have a desk in their bedroom and work late into the night. Others watch TV, snack, or eat meals in their bedroom. Others have a computer in the bedroom and find themselves surfing the Web into the early hours of the morning. All these behav-

> Many sleep problems are due to a disruptive sleep environment and to poor habits regarding time.

iors tend to be activating. They cause you to think about problems, opportunities, and projects. When you do energizing activities in your bedroom, it becomes a cue to feel alert, active, and busy rather than a cue for rest and sleep.

Your bedroom should be a place that is primarily associated with sleep. One of the first things you may need to do is move your other activities elsewhere. Watch TV in another room. Move your computer. Shift your desk to another room. Do your serious reading somewhere else. Your bedroom should become a room dedicated to sleep.

Decorate your bedroom in a manner that complements sleep. Soothing shades of blue, green, or off-white are more restful than bright or dark colors. Pictures of nature, a few plants, and graceful, simple curtains and furnishings can all make a bedroom pleasant and relaxing. You can even add a soothing fragrance such as lavender.

Bedroom Essentials

The most important part of the bedroom is the bed. But all too often the bed is a forgotten piece of equipment that is old, cheap, or second-hand. Because your bed is covered, it is easy to forget its condition and put up with whatever you have. In fact, if your mattress is more than ten years old, it is time to purchase a new one. And when it comes to buying a new mattress, you should aim to get the most comfortable one possible.

Your bedroom should be a place that is primarily associated with sleep.

A bigger mattress is better for a number of reasons. Most people change position from twelve to twenty-five times a night. If you have a narrow bed, you will feel cramped. If you sleep with another person, space is even more important. In a narrow bed, when your partner moves, he or she may inadvertently bump you, disturbing your sleep. And when one person moves, the other tends to move a few seconds later.

Mattresses typically come in the following sizes:

Twin	39" wide by 75" long
Double	54" wide by 75" long
Queen	60" wide by 75" long
King	76" wide by 80" long

A twin or a double-size mattress will suffice if you are sleeping alone, but a double is probably best. If you share your bed, a queen-size mattress is the minimum acceptable size. If you and your partner are big people, then get a king-size mattress. If you are tall, you can get an extra-long mattress eighty inches in length. Remember, don't skimp. A good mattress is an investment in your health.

Make sure your mattress is firm enough yet truly comfortable. Firmness in an innerspring mattress, the most

A good mattress is an investment in your health.

common kind of mattress, is determined by the thickness of the wire and the number of turns per coil. An inner-spring mattress is like a sandwich with steel springs in the middle, a layer of insulation on either side, and a cushion on the top and bottom. A high-quality mattress will have five to six turns per coil, a coil count of at least 720 coils per fifty-four square inches, thick insulation, and an outer cushion with some cotton so the material can breathe.

A good mattress should feel immediately relaxing and comfortable.

Beyond these technical considerations, the best way to determine if a mattress is going to be comfortable is to lie on it. A good mattress should feel immediately relaxing and comfortable. It should feel firm at the hips and shoulders. If you move or bounce, the mattress should absorb the pressure evenly. Purchase the matching box spring to get a unit designed to work together.

There are other kinds of mattresses, including foam pads and futons. Cheap, thin ones won't help your sleep. Thicker, better-quality pads and futons cost more but will help you sleep better. You can also add firmness to your current mattress by placing a sheet of plywood under it. You can add comfort to your mattress with a soft mattress pad.

Once you have a good mattress, then select a good pillow. Pillows serve the purpose of supporting your head, which makes up about 20 percent of your body weight.

When you lie on your side, a pillow can help your head to line up with your spine. People who sleep on their sides need the firmest pillows, while people who sleep on their backs or stomachs do fine with a softer pillow.

Then get the right sheets. The best measure of quality in sheets is thread count, which refers to the number of threads per square inch. Thread count can vary from 80 to 340. Sheets with a count of at least 180 to 200 and a plain weave are called *percale* and should give you satisfactory softness. Percale sheets come in 100 percent cotton or a cotton-polyester blend. Most people find that cotton is softer, breathes, and responds best to temperature changes. Flannel sheets can be wonderfully soft and warm in the winter.

Then select a blanket. Heavy blankets put weight on your chest and impede your breathing. Down comforters are very light and so warm that you can easily keep your bedroom cooler. A light cotton blanket may be all you need in the summer. Electric blankets are becoming more sophisticated and have zoned heat to provide more heat to your feet and less to your shoulders and chest.

Next, select comfortable bedclothes. Avoid anything tight or restrictive around the neck, ankles, or arms. Be aware of what feels most comfortable for you.

Electric blankets are becoming more sophisticated and have zoned heat to provide more heat to your feet and less to your shoulders and chest.

Light, Noise, and Temperature

Take a look around your bedroom and see what kind of light might be coming in. Common sources are streetlights, outside lights on your home, lights in other rooms, and even night-lights. Remember, the onset of darkness provides a daily signal to your biological clock that it is time to sleep. Light signals your inner clock that it is time to be awake and alert. Trying to sleep in a room with a lot of light sends your body a contradictory message. You want your bedroom to be dark.

Once you have identified sources of light, take steps to minimize them. First, turn out all the lights in your bedroom. If you feel you need a night-light in your house, position it outside your bedroom or have a motion sensor to turn it on. Curtains and shades can reduce any outside light. Blackout shades are also available, if you live in a well-lit area. A final option is to wear a soft pair of eyeshades.

Background noise can disrupt your sleep. Adults, particularly older adults, are more sensitive to noise than children. The problem comes when there is so much noise around us that we can never get complete, restful sleep.

Some background sounds can actually help us sleep. The steady patter of raindrops, leaves rustling in the wind, or the sound of ocean surf are all sounds that can lull us into a deep sleep. A common element of these sounds is that they are steady and rhythmic. It is the sudden, discordant,

Light signals your inner clock that it is time to be awake and alert.

irregular, and loud noises that trigger our protective alerting and disturb our sleep.

Assess the current noise levels in your bedroom. Are there disturbing sounds in your bedroom from a fan, a clock, or an old air conditioner? Are there disturbing noises in your home from a refrigerator, furnace, washer, dryer, or faucet? Does your partner snore or talk in his or her sleep? Are there noises outside your home from traffic, sirens, or factories?

Determine how many of the noises you can eliminate, reduce, or modify. You don't want to get neurotically obsessed with every little sound, but the general rule is the quieter your sleep environment, the better you will sleep.

Locate your bedroom in the quietest part of your home or apartment. Eliminate any unnecessary noise in your bedroom, such as ticking clocks. If you have a fan or an air conditioner, get a quality one that has a low frequency and a quiet, steady sound. If your pets make noises in your bedroom, it is time for them to sleep elsewhere. Try to get quiet appliances. You can reduce outside noise by having triple-pane windows and thick curtains and shades. Thick carpeting in your bedroom will also help absorb sound.

If you live in a noisy urban environment, you might need to block out all the sounds with the low hum of a fan or a quietly running air conditioner. You could also use a white-noise generator, a machine that emits sound contain-

Eliminate any unnecessary noise in your bedroom, such as ticking clocks.

Another alternative for blocking out sound is to use earplugs.

ing all the audible frequencies that effectively blocks out all other sounds. Tuning your TV or FM radio to an empty channel can provide you with a homemade white-noise machine. If you use a white-noise generator or environmental sounds, you probably want to program it to turn off after forty-five minutes because sometimes these sounds can prevent you from moving into deep sleep. Another alternative for blocking out sound is to use earplugs.

A final technique for dealing with a disturbing sound is to change your reaction. When noise from insects, trucks, or a nearby party prevents you from falling asleep, you will most likely focus on the noise and get more and more irritated and angry. Both these reactions are energizing and will make it harder to sleep. Breathe easily, try to appreciate and enjoy the sound, and just go with it. You can think of all the good the insects are doing, of the beautifully designed engines in the trucks and the things they are transporting. As you think positively and breathe easily, you can let go of your anger, relax into the sound, and drift off to sleep.

Temperature is another factor that influences sleep. Most people sleep best in a cooler environment with temperatures between sixty and seventy-two degrees. Remember, one of the physiological changes that goes with sleep is a drop in body temperature. A cooler room will help support this cycle. Sleeping in temperatures above seventy-five degrees may decrease the amount of slow wave and REM sleep you get.

Airflow is another factor that can make your bedroom more comfortable. Many people find it pleasant to open the windows and let some fresh air flow through the bedroom. If noise levels prevent that, then a quiet ceiling fan or room fan can help to circulate the air and keep it fresh.

Humidity can also influence your nighttime comfort. A dry room can dry out your nasal passages, creating an unpleasant feeling and making it harder to breathe at night. This is a common wintertime problem that contributes to the onset of colds. A humidifier will help to keep your air moister. On the other end of the spectrum, too much humidity is also uncomfortable. One of the great advantages of an air conditioner besides the cooler temperature is the reduced humidity.

Security is another factor to consider in making your bedroom a great place to sleep. If you don't feel safe and secure, you may find it difficult to fall asleep. Make sure you have a solid, strong door with an effective lock system and a dead bolt. A home security system or alarm system can offer you a greater sense of safety. Security lights with motion sensors outside your home can be helpful. The right breed of dog can also protect you at night, as long as it doesn't wake you up too often. Make sure you have a functioning smoke detector and a carbon monoxide detector as well.

A dry room can dry out your nasal passages, creating an unpleasant feeling and making it harder to breathe at night.

SETTING YOUR SLEEP SCHEDULE

Establishing a regular schedule and routine for your bedtime and wake-up time is one of the best things you can do for your sleep and for your overall health. When you have a regular sleep schedule, your inner clock can work efficiently so that at bedtime every aspect of your physiology is aligned to help you sleep. And when it is time to be alert, all levels of your body will be supporting this alertness. On the other hand, if you constantly go to bed and get up at different times, your inner clock is continually struggling to align your biorhythms.

Another important reason for having a regular sleep schedule is the force of habit. Humans have an innate capacity to learn habits—predictable automatic patterns of behavior. We don't have to struggle, decide, and start anew every day because the momentum of our habit carries us.

When we have a regular bedtime and a regular routine before bed, the whole process unfolds easily. One cue after another reminds us and prepares us for deep, restful sleep.

Sleep schedules and routines tend to be very individual and unique. Begin by looking at your natural tendencies. The self-assessment you conducted as part of Chapter 3 should have given you an idea of how much sleep you need and when you are naturally tired and alert. Take that information and combine it with the current reality factors in

When you have a regular sleep schedule, your inner clock can work efficiently so that at bedtime every aspect of your physiology is aligned to help you sleep.

your life regarding when you need to be at work, school, or awake to deal with family demands. Blending your natural preferences with your life demands should give you a good idea of what would be a suitable sleep schedule.

For example, if you need to wake up at 6 A.M. in order to be at work and you function best with seven hours of sleep, you would set your bedtime for no later than 11 P.M. But if you know that you naturally start to get tired at 10:30 P.M., then it makes sense to move your bedtime to 10:30 P.M. and get up a little earlier if you want.

Once you have determined a good sleep schedule, stick with it throughout the week. If you sleep late on Saturday and Sunday, you will find it hard to fall asleep at your regular bedtime Sunday night and then it will be even harder to get up early Monday morning. All this shifting of bedtime and wake-up time plays havoc with your inner clock and sleep system.

Of course, your sleep system is designed to be resilient. If you need to or choose to stay up late, that's fine. Just get your core sleep of five to six hours, get up as close as possible to your normal wake-up time, and work off the sleep debt during the next night. But strive to adopt and maintain a regular sleep schedule.

Wind-Down Time
Once you have established your ideal bedtime, carve out

> Blending your natural preferences and your life demands should give you a good idea of what would be a suitable sleep schedule.

One of the biggest mistakes people make is to work right up to their bedtime.

about thirty to sixty minutes before your bedtime as sleep preparation time, or wind-down time. One of the biggest mistakes people make is to work right up to their bedtime. These undertakings are activating, they engage us in planning, thinking, and even worrying. When we are activated, it is harder to fall asleep.

Stop working, studying, paying bills, talking on the phone, or playing computer games. Omit any serious television-watching such as documentaries, hard news shows, or violence. In other words, simply omit things that are activating and energizing or that cause worries or concerns.

Don't eat in the hour before bedtime. Avoid sugary food that will raise your blood sugar. Avoid spicy foods that might cause indigestion or heartburn. Avoid high-protein foods that are usually energizing.

When it comes to adding things, you will find it very helpful to do a few stretches to release any muscular tension that has built up during the day. Or you can do a brief session of relaxation. A routine of stretching exercises as well as relaxation techniques will be presented in the next chapter.

A hot bath or shower can be another helpful component of a wind-down routine. The warm water will directly relax your muscles. You will feel refreshed and cleansed from the day's concerns. And a hot bath will temporarily raise your body temperature. As your body cools down, you will feel sleepy, just as you naturally feel sleepy when your body cools down at night.

There are many other activities that can be part of a wind-down routine. You may find it relaxing to listen to soothing music. You may find that certain kinds of reading, such as travel books, romances, or adventures, can help you get your mind off things and relax.

Look for things that help you slow down and prepare yourself for sleep. Find things that work, and stick to them so you establish an enjoyable wind-down routine that you look forward to every night. From time to time, add new things to your routine to keep it fresh and interesting.

Look for things that help you slow down and prepare yourself for sleep.

Your Bedtime Routine

Once you have gone through your wind-down time, you should be ready to start your bedtime routine, a series of specific steps that gradually and certainly leads you to fall easily into a sound sleep. This routine typically starts with a phase of shutting down your living environment for the night. This could include such steps as shutting the windows, closing the doors, locking up, adjusting the thermostat, and turning out lights.

The next phase has to do with your physical preparation for bed. Change into your sleeping clothes. Begin a personal grooming routine that includes flossing and brushing your teeth, washing your face, applying lotion, and brushing your hair.

The final part of your bedtime routine will involve actually getting into bed. You might do a few last stretches, climb into bed, pull up the covers, read for a few minutes, and then turn out the lights. At this point in your bedtime routine, you will be ready to switch to what might be called your sleep-time routine. You will be ready to do some of the relaxation and breathing techniques to be described in the following chapters.

Your Wake-Up Routine

There are a number of ways a wake-up routine can help you. First of all, a regular routine will simply make it easier to get up and get started. Just as a sleep routine makes it easier to fall asleep, a wake-up routine makes it easier to get up.

A second benefit from a wake-up routine is that it can help reset your biological clock. When you wake up and take in sunlight, it recalibrates your inner clock which in turn helps you to maintain a regular sleep-and-alertness pattern. And remember that as soon as you wake up, you are beginning to accumulate the sleep debt you need to help you sleep at night. A routine that helps you get up early is strengthening your daily sleep cycle.

Wake-up routines are likely to be influenced by your

When you wake up and take in sunlight, it recalibrates your inner clock which in turn helps you to maintain a regular sleep-and-alertness pattern.

personal taste, living situation, and schedule demands. Most people have a routine developed more by accident than design. Now you can design a routine that is beneficial. It doesn't need to be long if you are pressed for time. Even a five-minute routine can be helpful.

When you wake up, the first thing to do is to simply notice and take in the light. Let some natural light enter your eyes and welcome you into the day.

Next you might tune yourself to a positive emotional state. Think of some things that you can look forward to. It might be your breakfast, the people you will share the day with, a place you will see, work you will do, or something you will learn.

When you get out of bed, you most likely will start some kind of bathroom routine. After elimination you might want to wash your hands and face and brush your teeth. You might want to jump into a nice hot shower.

Because your body is stiff when you wake up, some form of exercise is often a very beneficial part of a wake-up routine. You can start by doing a few loosening stretches in bed. Wiggle your fingers and toes. Move your wrists and ankles. Point your toes away and stretch your legs. Straighten your arms. This will help to loosen your muscles and raise your body temperature.

Some people like to do a more intensive exercise session to start the day. This might involve a session of yoga. It

Because your body is stiff when you wake up, some form of exercise is often a very beneficial part of a wake-up routine.

might involve weight-lifting, aerobics, running, walking, biking, or swimming.

Another option is to start the day with a spiritual practice such as meditation, contemplation, prayer, or scripture reading. Or begin by devoting some time to artistic or creative undertakings such as writing, drawing, or painting.

There are many enjoyable and healthy components you can bring into your wake-up routine. The key point is that you start the day with energy and set the stage for a daytime routine of being alert, getting exercise, and getting some exposure to natural light throughout the day.

Start the day with energy and set the stage for a daytime routine of being alert, getting exercise, and getting some exposure to natural light throughout the day.

Time for Sex

Bedtime is the time that many couples have sex. For a lot of people, this works great. They feel peaceful and relaxed after making love. They forget about all their worries. They feel emotionally close, loved, and satisfied. After making love, they find it easy to drift into a deep, satisfying sleep. If this is the case for you and your partner, then sex can be a beneficial part of your bedtime routine.

There are several circumstances when lovemaking can interfere with sleep. Some people find sex very activating. After making love they feel alert and energized and would have a hard time falling asleep. For such individuals, having sex earlier in the day would be better.

The second problem scenario comes when a couple is

experiencing conflict about sex or if one or both partners has some sexual dysfunction. In such cases, sex may bring up worry, anxiety, or even anger. These feelings tend to be activating and to interfere with sleep onset and quality. In this situation, a couple may need to work out their differences with the help of a sex therapist.

TIME AND ENVIRONMENT

There are three key points in choices about time and environment. The first is that you are taking an active role in improving your sleep. You are not just going through patterns that developed accidentally, but choosing what is best for your well-being.

The second point is that you are giving sleep the priority it deserves in your life. Instead of squeezing sleep in as an afterthought, you are making it a true priority.

The third point is that you are making sleep truly pleasant and enjoyable, which it should be. Sleep is one of the real blessings and pleasures of life. When you make sleep a priority and create a comfortable and optimal sleep environment, you will once again enjoy sleep.

Instead of squeezing sleep in as an afterthought, you are making it a true priority.

preparing your body for sleep: reducing muscular tension

Sleep is sweet to the laboring man.

John Bunyan

M uscular tension is one of the biggest obstacles to falling asleep. Recall the times you have climbed into bed wanting to fall asleep and found that you just couldn't get comfortable. Perhaps you noticed tightness in your neck and shoulders or even had a headache or a sore back. Or maybe your body was so wired for action that you couldn't calm down and go to sleep. These are all symptoms of muscular tension.

On the other hand, remember a day when you took a long walk or went cross-country skiing. After exercise and fresh air, you felt so relaxed that you fell asleep immediately. Or you had a long bath or even a massage. Your muscles were completely relaxed. You fell quickly asleep.

To experience complete natural sleep, we need to learn how to let go of muscular tension. As a first step, we need to understand how the muscles work.

THE MUSCULAR SYSTEM

There are three types of muscles. *Cardiac muscles* in the heart maintain a rhythmic contraction to pump blood through the body. *Smooth muscles* are found in the internal organs such as the stomach and intestines. But our concern is with the *skeletal muscles* that connect to the bones and cross the joints. These are the muscles beneath the surface of the skin that allow us to stand and move. The skeletal muscles make up 40 to 50 percent of our body weight.

An example of a skeletal muscle is the biceps, between your elbow and your shoulder on the inside of your arm. The biceps is made up of numerous muscle fibers. A small group of fibers is controlled by a single nerve known as a *motor neuron.* The motor neuron emerges from the spinal cord and branches out at its end to connect with a number of muscle fibers. When the motor neuron is activated, the muscle fibers contract. Motor units fire in a synchronous manner, creating a smooth muscle contraction.

The motor units are controlled by a part of the brain known as the *sensory motor cortex.* This part of the brain can contract a single muscle when we move a finger or can orchestrate a pattern of muscular activation to produce such complex movements as walking or running. As well as sending out signals to activate the muscles, the sensory motor cortex also receives sensory information coming in from the muscles. If a muscle becomes tired or is in pain, that information is relayed immediately to the brain.

Chronic muscular tension is created when there is a breakdown in the communication and teamwork between the muscles and the brain. Tension means that muscles

Chronic muscular tension is created when there is a breakdown in the communication and teamwork between the muscles and the brain.

remain contracted and tight. This may be caused by constant overactivation. The brain, in response to some stressful demand, keeps activating the muscles. This combination of sustained contraction and limited awareness can create a cycle of ever increasing muscular tension that interferes with a good night's sleep.

THE CAUSES OF MUSCULAR TENSION

Constant, repetitive contraction of specific groups of muscles is one of the major causes of muscular tension. This occurs when we repeat a certain position over and over. For example, if we sit at a desk working on a computer all day, we are flexing the muscles of our back and extending our neck forward. Along with these postural demands, we may be tightening the muscles across the forehead and around the eyes as we concentrate. We may be tightening our jaw muscles as we "bite" into our work. We may be bracing our legs as we "race" to meet a deadline.

After a few hours, our muscles are locked into a pattern of tension and we are so absorbed with our work that we don't even notice the signals of protest coming from our muscles. If we stand up and do a few stretches, we suddenly realize how much tension we have been holding.

Constant, repetitive contraction of specific groups of muscles is one of the major causes of muscular tension.

Unfortunately, most of us don't take a break.

Over time, all the sitting and leaning and bracing can lead to chronic tension. Tightness accumulates in the neck and back. The muscles begin to adapt and shorten, locking us into a pattern of tension.

A sedentary lifestyle is another cause of muscular tension.

Another cause of muscular tension is constant overactivation. Many people rush around from daybreak to midnight. The day starts with the jarring ring of the alarm clock. Then the morning scramble starts, rushing to get showered and dressed, herding the kids to the school bus, and then jumping into the car to do battle with the traffic. During the workday there is constant hurrying, sitting, talking, and thinking. The afternoon traffic battle sets the stage for an evening of dinner, cleanup, kids' homework, and jobs around the house.

All day long we have been relentlessly firing up the muscles. Each task, each deadline, each confrontation causes a little more tightness in the shoulders, neck, back, and across the face. We are so focused on the things we need to do that we ignore the accumulating tension. But when we get in bed at night and try to sleep, we feel like a coiled spring. Even if we feel tired, we just can't let go of all the muscular tension.

A sedentary lifestyle is another cause of muscular tension. When we are active, we contract the muscles forcefully, and at the end of the activity or exercise the muscles naturally relax. If we are inactive and sit around most of the time, our muscles never have the opportunity to release tension in a natural fashion.

Another cause of muscular tension is strong negative emotions. Stressful situations that cause flashes of anger, fear, or anxiety set off the primitive and powerful "flight or fight" response that is quickly translated into muscular activation. With fear, our muscles are braced to flee, and with anger, our muscles are primed to fight. With anxiety, our body tightens up with vigilance. With sadness, we frown, tightening the muscles around our eyes.

We experience these emotions throughout the day. The problem is that we rarely express the underlying impetus for movement and action. We hold a strategic poker face over seething anger. We exude calmness to cover fear and anxiety. We force a smile to cover our sadness. But the emotions and their associated muscular activations remain and are turned into muscular tension that builds and builds.

Muscular tension from all these causes creates a self-perpetuating system. The tension never gets released. Every day we add to our store of tension. Every day it gets harder to relax our muscles.

Another cause of muscular tension is strong negative emotions.

The Effects of Muscular Tension on Sleep

Muscular tension is part of the human activation response. This activation response is the direct opposite of sleep.

When we are tense, we just can't fall asleep. The tense, activated muscles urge the brain to stay alert and awake. It is very difficult to shift from this active state to sleep. Muscular tension also makes it hard to get comfortable. Sometimes muscular tension causes a headache or a backache. This pain makes it even harder to fall asleep.

When people who are tense wake up during the night, they often have a harder time falling back asleep.

It takes energy to tighten the muscles. If we are tensed up, we are using extra energy. We will feel worn out and tired, but paradoxically this same tension makes it hard to fall asleep and get the rest we crave.

Tension persists throughout the night and interferes with the quality of sleep. Tense people get less deep sleep. When people who are tense wake up during the night, they often have a harder time falling back asleep. They wake up feeling stiff and tired. To get complete sleep, we need to break the cycle of muscular tension.

PRINCIPLES OF MUSCULAR RELAXATION

Muscular relaxation is a skill that can be learned through instruction and practice. We need to be aware of the signals going out from the brain tensing up the muscles, and we need to be aware of the feedback coming from the muscles. Once we have awareness, we can learn control techniques to actively reduce unnecessary and harmful tension.

Types of Muscular Relaxation

There are two broad approaches to muscular relaxation: conscious relaxation, and exercise. Conscious relaxation involves learning to directly decrease the level of activation in the muscles. With exercise, muscular relaxation follows exertion. A long walk or vigorous workout leaves you feeling relaxed and peaceful.

The Basic Relaxation Posture

The best position for practicing conscious relaxation is to lie down on your back on a padded carpet. Bring your legs together and bring your arms alongside your body. Align your body so that you have a straight line from your nose to your chin to your navel down to your big toes. Then move your legs out eight inches away from this center line and move your arms about eight inches away from your torso. Open your hands and let your palms face upward.

This basic relaxation posture is known as *Shavasana* in the tradition of hatha yoga. Shavasana means "corpse pose," the idea being that when you practice this relaxation posture, you shed your tense, stressed-out body to be reborn with a relaxed and refreshed body.

Before you settle into this basic relaxation posture, make sure you are comfortable. Wear loose clothing. Take off your glasses. Remove your belt, watch, and any tight or

The best position for practicing conscious relaxation is to lie down on your back on a padded carpet.

constricting jewelry. If your lower back is stiff, you might be more comfortable with a pillow under your knees. Try to select a quiet room where you will be free from interruptions. Make sure the room isn't too chilly, because you will cool down as you relax. But if the room is too warm, you might drift off to sleep. If you can't stretch out on the floor, then select a comfortable chair.

The Practice of Differential Relaxation

Differential relaxation is a technique that trains you to become fully aware of the process of tensing and relaxing specific muscle groups. When you practice this technique, you will tense or activate the muscles on one side of the body and at the same time release and relax the muscles on the other side of the body. For example, as you tense the muscles in your right arm, you will relax the muscles in your left arm.

The key terms with this method are "active" and "passive." As you make one set of muscles active, you make the other set passive. Hold the activation for about ten seconds and release for about fifteen to twenty seconds. This method teaches you to become more attuned to the sensations of tension and relaxation in the muscles. At the same time, you will become increasingly aware of the systems in the brain that control muscular tension. With practice, you will become adept at using this control system to com-

Differential relaxation teaches you to become more attuned to the sensations of tension and relaxation in the muscles.

pletely let go of muscular tension throughout your body.

Differential relaxation is a very effective relaxation method, particularly for people beginning to learn relaxation. Because it is an active step-by-step process, it keeps you involved and focused on the process of relaxation. The CD accompanying this book contains a guided session of differential relaxation.

Differential relaxation is an ideal method to use during your wind-down time before bed. It will help you let go of the cares of the day and feel comfortable and ready for sleep. Differential relaxation can also be used at the end of a session of stretching exercises and during the day or after work to let go of tension and establish relaxation.

Guided Relaxation

Guided relaxation is a mentally directed approach to muscular relaxation. Instead of physically tensing and releasing the muscles, you simply bring your attention to specific muscle groups and direct the muscles to relax. Typically you start with the feet and work all the way up to your forehead.

This technique works best after you have had training and gained experience in differential relaxation. You need to develop a good sense of where the muscle groups are in your body, how to recognize unnecessary tension in those muscles, and how to direct them to relax. You also have to be able to maintain your focus as you move your awareness

Differential relaxation is a very effective relaxation method, particularly for people beginning to learn relaxation.

through the various muscle groups.

Guided relaxation can be practiced as part of your wind-down routine, after exercise, or during the day. It is also very well suited to be part of your sleep-time routine, meaning that after you get into bed, you can go through a guided relaxation to completely relax your muscles and make it easy to drift off to sleep. A session of guided relaxation is on the CD accompanying this book.

Exercise

Exercise helps to release the muscular tension that accumulates from repeated fight-or-flight responses. Most forms of exercise are socially appropriate ways of expressing this locked-up fighting-and-fleeing potential.

The fleeing exercises include walking, running, swimming, biking, cross-country skiing, rowing, ice skating, and even in-line skating. Exercises that express the trapped urge to fight typically involve some element of struggle, such as occurs with weight lifting. Competitive sports such as tennis or volleyball allow for socially approved expressions of aggression. After a good contest most people feel relaxed, particularly if they can cultivate a balance between playing hard and enjoying the activity.

Martial arts, such as karate and judo, provide another constructive approach to channeling and expressing fighting energy. The routines, or *katas*, of karate, with their

Guided relaxation can be practiced as part of your wind-down routine, after exercise, or during the day.

elements of punching, kicking, and blocking, provide a direct but disciplined expression of aggression.

Exercise and Good Sleep

When you have exercised during the day, you simply feel more like resting at night—you feel naturally tired, you sleep better at night, and you then are more inclined to be active the next day. Exercise and sleep complement each other.

Exercise also reduces muscular tension. It helps with sleep by temporarily raising our temperature. One cause of sleep difficulties is an inadequate or irregular temperature cycle. When we run, bike, or lift weights, our body temperature rises. Later when our temperature drops, we are more inclined to sleep.

The Practice of Exercise

The good news about exercise is that it doesn't take a lot to make a huge difference. Even walking as little as one mile three to five times a week can help you reap the benefits of exercise.

Accordingly, the first principle in bringing exercise into your life is to start modestly. Set a goal that fits your physical capacity as well as your time budget.

The second and perhaps most important principle is consistency. Exercise at least three to five times a week.

When you have exercised during the day, you simply feel more like resting at night—you feel naturally tired.

Make a commitment.

But also make the exercise fun and rewarding. If you choose walking, find a pleasant place to walk. If possible, pick a time that is pleasing. If you exercise inside, make your surroundings pleasant, listen to music, or watch videos. Make your exercise interesting. Incorporate variety. Walk or run in different places. On different days swim or bike. Exercise with other people and by yourself.

Two things will help you sustain your exercise routine. The first is enjoyment. If you find your exercise fun, pleasant, and rewarding, you will be motivated to do it. Awareness is the second great motivator. When you notice the tension melting, when you feel the increased energy, when you observe your mind becoming clearer and your emotions more peaceful and positive, when you notice you are sleeping better, you will want to exercise.

Don't participate in strenuous exercise too close to your scheduled sleep time. Exercise can be physically energizing, have an alerting effect, and raise your body temperature. Both effects could interfere with falling asleep. A good guideline is to complete your active exercise at least an hour or two before you begin your wind-down routine.

Stretching Exercises

Another way to release the muscular tension that builds up through the day is through stretching. With this type of exer-

A good guideline is to complete your active exercise at least an hour or two before you begin your wind-down routine.

cise, instead of acting out or vigorously expressing the trapped tension, you loosen and lengthen the muscles, thereby releasing the tension. Stretching exercises improve circulation, enhance flexibility, and create a feeling of well-being.

Stretching exercises actually involve the interaction of opposing groups of muscles. For example, if you bend your hand back, you are contracting the muscles on top of your lower arm and stretching the muscles on the bottom of your lower arm. Activating one muscle of a pair automatically inhibits activity in the other, allowing it to stretch.

Stretching Exercises and Sleep

Stretching exercises can be a very helpful part of your winddown or bedtime routine. If you spend a lot of time during the day sitting, driving, leaning forward to talk, or working on a computer, you will inevitably accumulate tension in your neck, shoulders, and back.

If you take fifteen to thirty minutes to perform some stretches before bed, you can get rid of most of this tension. When you stretch the tension out of your muscles, worries seem to disappear and you feel more peaceful. And after a series of stretching exercises, you will feel so comfortable and relaxed that once you get in bed you will naturally fall asleep.

Stretching exercises are a nice complement to active exercise. During active exercise, you vigorously express the

Stretching exercises are a nice complement to active exercise.

trapped activation in your body. But with stretching exercises, you loosen specific knots of tension.

Stretching exercises are convenient in that they can be performed close to bedtime without any risk of activating or stimulating the mind and body. Stretching exercises are also very practical. On a busy day when you don't get a chance to go running or walking, a series of stretching exercises can help you relax before bedtime. If the weather is bad or you are traveling, you can still do a routine of stretching exercises to release muscular tension.

The Practice of Stretching Exercises

Proceed gently when you practice stretching exercises. Stretch easily. Avoid any bouncing or pushing. If you attempt to stretch a muscle past its comfortable capacity, you will elicit the stretch reflex—when the muscle contracts to protect itself. This will ruin any chance of relaxation. Another guideline is to avoid pain. As soon as you feel any resistance or discomfort, don't stretch any further.

Stretching exercises are most effective when you coordinate your breathing with the stretches. Don't hold your breath as you stretch. Instead, breathe evenly and smoothly as you go into the stretch. Then with each exhalation, ease a little further into the stretch. As you integrate breathing and stretching, you will rapidly erase chronic tension, become more flexible, and be well prepared to sleep at night.

As you integrate breathing and stretching, you will rapidly erase chronic tension, become more flexible, and be well prepared to sleep at night.

Here is a series of stretching exercises designed to address most of the major muscle groups in the body, with particular emphasis on the neck, shoulders, chest, and upper back, regions where tension often accumulates. With most of these exercises you will hold the stretch for ten seconds and repeat it three times. As mentioned above, proceed gently. Bring your full awareness to the exercises. Breathe evenly and smoothly as you stretch. Don't watch TV and stretch. A quiet room with soothing music creates a good environment. Wear loose, comfortable clothing. Remove any constricting ties, belts, or jewelry.

A quiet room with soothing music creates a good environment for stretching.

1. **Overhead Stretch**
    Stand with your feet shoulder-width apart. Reach your arms straight up from your shoulders with your palms facing each other. Stretch up from your legs, through your torso, into your shoulders, arms, and hands. Hold for ten seconds. Then bring your arms back down. Inhale as you stretch up, breathe evenly as you hold, and exhale as you bring your arms down. Repeat two more times.

2. **Neck Exercises**
    Standing, with your back straight, bring your head forward, chin toward your chest. Hold for three seconds and tilt your neck back for three seconds. Go as far as

you can without creating any discomfort. Then slowly rotate your head to the right, chin over your right shoulder. Stretch as far as you comfortably can. Hold for three seconds. Then rotate your head to the left for three seconds. Tilt your head so your right ear comes down toward your right shoulder. Hold that for three seconds and then tilt your head to the left for three seconds. Repeat all three stretches two more times. Breathe smoothly during the neck stretches.

3. **Shoulder Stretch**
   With your fingers interlaced behind your back, straighten your arms and turn your elbows in until you feel the stretch. Hold for ten seconds. Breathe evenly. Repeat two more times.

4. **Rotator Cuff–Extensor Stretch**
   Either sitting on your heels or standing, bring your left hand, with the palm facing out, as far up your back as you can. Then reach your right hand back to join your left hand. Breathe evenly and hold the stretch for ten seconds. Reverse the position of your hands, and hold that for ten seconds. Do three repetitions. This very beneficial stretch can be difficult at first. Beginners can use a belt. Grasp the belt with both hands and gradually work the hands closer together.

5. **Chest Stretch**

   Clasp your hands behind your head. Stretch your elbows back. Hold for ten seconds and breathe evenly. Repeat two more times.

6. **Biceps Stretch**

   Clasp your hands behind your back. Straighten your arms and lift up until you feel the stretch in your chest and arms. Hold for ten seconds. Breathe evenly. Repeat two more times.

7. **Hand and Wrist Stretch**

   Bring your arms in front of your body. Interlace your fingers with your palms facing out. Straighten your arms until you feel the stretch in your lower arms and wrists. Breathe evenly while you hold for ten seconds. Repeat two more times.

8. **Hip Stretch**

   Stand with your feet together and your arms straight over your head with the palms touching. Bend to the right, feeling the stretch on the left side of your body. Hold for ten seconds. Breathe evenly as you stretch. In the same way, bend to the left. Repeat two more times to each side.

9. **Trunk Rotation**

   Stand with your feet shoulder-width apart. Rotate your trunk to the right, leading with your extended left arm. Bring your right arm behind your back. Hold for ten seconds. Breathe evenly at the point of stretch. Then rotate to the left, reversing the position of your arms. Repeat two more times.

10. **Hamstring Stretch**

    Standing, place your right heel on a chair or bench. Support yourself by placing your hands on your right upper leg. Keep your torso straight and bend forward until you feel the stretch. Hold for ten seconds. Breathe evenly. Do the same stretch with the left leg. Repeat two more times.

11. **Upper Leg Stretch**

    Rest your left hand on a chair or table for balance. Grab your right foot with your right hand and pull your heel toward your buttock until you feel the stretch. Hold for ten seconds, breathing evenly. Repeat with the other leg. Do two more stretches for each leg.

12. **Calf Stretch**

    Bring your left foot forward, bending the knee. Place your right foot back with your heel flat on the floor.

Bend down on your left leg while contracting the thigh muscles of your right leg. Feel the stretch in your calf muscles. Breathe evenly and hold for ten seconds. Reverse the position and stretch your left calf. Repeat two more times on each side.

13. Integration Posture

Cross your right leg over and place your right foot to the left of your left foot. Cross your left wrist over your right and interlace your fingers. Bring your arms down and then pull your joined hands up to your chest. Hold for fifteen seconds, breathing evenly. Release the position. Then cross your left leg over, placing your left foot to the right of your right foot. Cross your right wrist over your left, interlace your fingers, bring your arms down, and then pull your joined hands up to your chest. Hold and breathe evenly for fifteen seconds.

When you have completed this routine of stretches, you should feel much looser. If the stretches are an early step in your wind-down routine, you may want to follow them by doing a differential or guided relaxation. If the stretches are the last step in your wind-down routine, you can move right into your bedtime and sleep-time routines. With your muscles loose and flexible, you should feel comfortable and relaxed when you get into bed, ready to drift off to sleep.

With your muscles loose and flexible, you should feel comfortable and relaxed when you get into bed, ready to easily drift off to sleep.

overcoming inner tension: the autonomic nervous system

Sweet is the breath of morn, her rising sweet,
with charm of earliest birds.

John Milton, *Paradise Lost*

E ven when your muscles are relaxed, you may find that you still feel too restless to fall asleep. You may notice that your heart is beating too fast, your breath is too shallow and rapid, your stomach is tied in knots, and your hands feel cold and clammy. These are all signs of inner tension triggered by the autonomic nervous system.

It may seem like there is no way to slow your heart and calm your stomach. But once you understand how the autonomic nervous system works and learn effective methods of autonomic relaxation, you will be able to calm this inner turbulence and obtain complete, natural sleep.

This inner tension, while more subtle than muscular tension, can be just as harmful to sleep.

THE AUTONOMIC NERVOUS SYSTEM

The autonomic nervous system (ANS) is designed to create the inner mobilization to accompany and support the fight-or-flight response. At the moment we brace our muscles to fight or flee, the ANS raises our heart rate, increases our blood pressure, and shuts down our digestion. All this happens instantly and without any conscious decision.

The ANS has two branches: *sympathetic* and *parasym-*

pathetic. It is the sympathetic branch that activates the body for the fight-or-flight response. When this part of the ANS remains activated, it is hard to fall asleep. The parasympathetic branch decreases inner activation and moves the body to a rest-and-housekeeping mode that can support sleep.

The Sympathetic Branch of the ANS

The nerves of the sympathetic branch leave the spinal column from the neck down to the lower back, as seen in Figure 1. These fibers travel to the major internal organs, including the heart, lungs, stomach, adrenal gland, kidneys, intestine, and anal sphincter. Sympathetic nerves also reach out to the sweat glands and blood vessels in the periphery of the body and control the piloerector muscles that make the hair on our arms stand up when we are afraid or angry.

Sympathetic activation supports the fight-or-flight response in a number of ways. Increased heart rate prepares the body for action. Constriction of the blood vessels in the hands and feet moves more blood to the heart and brain and lessens blood flow to the hands or feet to protect the body in case of injury to the extremities. Sympathetic activa-

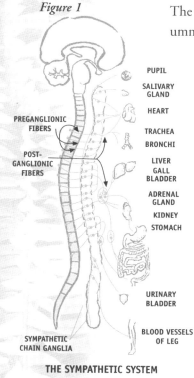

Figure 1

PREGANGLIONIC FIBERS

POST-GANGLIONIC FIBERS

PUPIL
SALIVARY GLAND
HEART
TRACHEA
BRONCHI
LIVER
GALL BLADDER
ADRENAL GLAND
KIDNEY
STOMACH

URINARY BLADDER

SYMPATHETIC CHAIN GANGLIA

BLOOD VESSELS OF LEG

THE SYMPATHETIC SYSTEM

tion shuts down digestion and slows peristalsis. Breathing rate increases. Basal metabolism goes up and glucose is released into the bloodstream. The adrenal gland releases hormones that enhance and sustain the stress response. Mentally, sympathetic activation creates a very alert, vigilant, and active state. But when this activation is maintained for too long, it can stress the heart, elevate blood p
cause digestive problems, deplete energy, and c
interfere with falling asleep.

The Parasympathetic Branch of the ANS

The parasympathetic branch of the ANS has a different structure. Nerves emerge from the brain stem and the sacral area of the spine. As shown in Figure 2, the parasympathetic branch affects many of the same organs as the sympathetic branch. But the parasympathetic branch creates a very different internal state. The parasympathetic branch slows things so the body can rest, rebuild, and heal.

Specifically, the parasympathetic branch acts to slow heart rate and decrease blood pressure. Breathing slows and deepens. Peristalsis is increased and digestion improved. Metabolism slows. The gallbladder, liver, and bladder are stimulated to perform their housekeeping

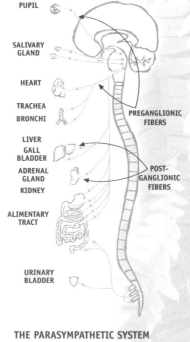

THE PARASYMPATHETIC SYSTEM

tasks. Mentally, parasympathetic activation is associated with a calm, peaceful state.

Excessive parasympathetic activation can slow things down too much. Excessive slowing is often associated with feelings of helplessness and despair. People caught in this pattern may actually sleep too much.

The ANS is designed to deal with infrequent but life-threatening emergencies.

Patterns of Autonomic Tension

Ideally, the two branches of the autonomic nervous system should interact in a complementary fashion. The sympathetic branch activates our inner resources to deal with a threat; when it is over, parasympathetic activation slows things so we can rebuild our inner resources.

Autonomic tension occurs when we lose this healthy balance. The most common pattern of autonomic imbalance is excessive sympathetic activation. This is associated with such destructive stress disorders as heart disease, hypertension, digestive problems, and sleep difficulties.

One reason for this excessive sympathetic activation may lie in the makeup of the ANS. This system is designed to deal with infrequent but life-threatening emergencies. The rest of the time, parasympathetic activation supports rest and recovery.

But the tempo of modern life influences sympathetic activation. Instead of an occasional emergency, we face a constant attack of low-level stressors. Sympathetic activation is turned on during the morning commute and stays on throughout the workday. We live with constant low-grade sympathetic activation.

Another cause of excessive sympathetic activation is persistent negative emotions. Strong feelings such as anger, fear, and anxiety instantly cause sympathetic activation. When we are afraid, the ANS triggers an increase in heart beat, rapid shallow breath, and sweaty palms. When we are so angry that we "see red," it is the ANS that orchestrates the rising blood pressure and shaky feelings inside.

Anytime we have strong emotions, we have an autonomic response. Many of us live with persistent feelings of anger, fear, and anxiety. We feel angry about our job, relationships, neighbors, and traffic. We fear for our safety and security. We feel anxious about finances and the future. These feelings lead to excessive sympathetic activation.

Anytime we have strong emotions, we have an autonomic response.

Excessive parasympathetic activation is another type of autonomic tension. In this case there is too much inhibition. This leads to a lack of energy, slowed digestion, and inadequate breathing. This imbalance is linked to such negative emotions as sadness, hopelessness, and despair.

The Impact of ANS Tension on Sleep

When we have excessive sympathetic activation, it is hard to fall asleep. An elevated heart rate and increased blood pressure are part of an alert state. This state is diametrically opposed to sleep. Consequently, when we go to bed with excessive sympathetic activation, we will lie there but feel so wired we simply can't let go and drift off to sleep.

And if and when we do finally fall asleep, the quality of our sleep will be poor. If we go to sleep feeling agitated, we will be restless through the night. We may wake up more frequently and have more difficulty falling back asleep. And if we go to sleep with ANS tension, we may find that when we get up in the morning, we don't feel rested because we never fully shifted our body to the rest-and-recovery mode.

On the other hand, if we have excessive parasympathetic responding, we may find it difficult to get up and get started in the morning. We won't have the energy to rise early and jump into our wake-up routine. And if we sleep too late, we are likely to disrupt our sleep schedule so we have even more difficulty falling asleep the next night.

If we have both kinds of ANS tension, we are in the doubly difficult position of struggling to fall asleep, sleeping poorly, and then struggling to get up in the morning. ANS tension can have a very harmful effect on sleep.

Breathing and Autonomic Relaxation

The autonomic nervous system may seem difficult to relax. The very name *autonomic* seems to infer that this system runs on its own. And certainly it is hard to imagine consciously decreasing heart rate and dropping blood pressure.

If we go to sleep feeling agitated, we will be restless through the night.

There are several things we can use to rebalance and relax the ANS. The first of these is the breath. There is a reciprocal relationship between the breath and the ANS.

There are four aspects of breathing that interact with the ANS: form, rate, ratio of inhalation to exhalation, and smoothness of the breath. *Form* refers to the mechanics of how we move the air in and out of our lungs. In this regard, there are three types of breath, each associated with a distinct pattern of ANS activation.

The first type is *clavicular breathing*, where you lift the shoulders when you inhale and drop them when you exhale. This is an inefficient type of breathing used only during moments of crisis or when we are having difficulty getting air in. Clavicular breathing is associated with strong sympathetic activation.

The most common type of breathing is *thoracic*, where we lift and expand the chest with inhalation and bring the chest down and in with exhalation. While this type of breathing is more efficient than clavicular, it is directly associated with sympathetic activation. Thoracic breathing is part of the fight-or-flight response. The motion of the lungs in thoracic breathing directly stimulates sympathetic activation, increasing heart rate and blood pressure. If you are breathing thoracically when you go to bed, it will be difficult to fall asleep.

The third type of breathing is called *diaphragmatic*.

There is a reciprocal relationship between the breath and the ANS.

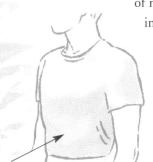

EXHALE

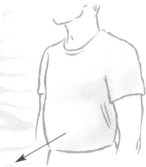

INHALE

With this type of breathing, the diaphragm, a strong layer of muscles underneath the lungs, works with the abdominal muscles. When you exhale, you contract the abdominal muscles and pull them in. At the same time, the diaphragm relaxes and moves up in a dome, pushing the old air out of the lungs. When you relax your abdominal muscles, the diaphragm contracts down, expanding the chest cavity and allowing fresh air to flow in.

Diaphragmatic breathing is very efficient in terms of cleaning old air out of the lungs and bringing fresh air deep into the lungs for optimal oxygenation of the blood. Most importantly, the motion of the lungs during diaphragmatic breathing has a direct influence on the ANS to decrease sympathetic activation. Diaphragmatic breathing is associated with a mentally quiet and emotionally calm state and in every way is more conducive to falling asleep.

Rate is the second dimension of breathing linked to the ANS. A person locked into a simmering fight-or-flight response is likely to breathe twenty to thirty breaths per minute. In a state of ANS relaxation, the breathing rate will slow to a calm and comfortable eight to twelve breaths per minute. The slower breathing rate will be much more conducive to sleep.

Within a single breath, inhalation is associated with sympathetic activation while exhalation is associated with parasympathetic activation. The individual who is anxious and stressed out will be inhaling strenuously, while the person who is caught up in hopelessness and depression will emit long, sighing exhalations. Autonomic relaxation occurs when inhalation and exhalation are in *balance*.

Autonomic relaxation is also associated with s*moothly* flowing breath that courses from inhalation to exhalation and back in a graceful wave. Autonomic tension is associated with pauses in the breath: when we hold our breath in fear or anger, or when we pause after a long, sad exhalation.

These four aspects of breath can be used to create autonomic relaxation. If you can consciously establish even, smooth, slow, diaphragmatic breathing, you will experience autonomic relaxation and be ready for sleep.

THE PRACTICE OF DIAPHRAGMATIC BREATHING

The CD accompanying this book contains a guided practice of diaphragmatic breathing. Here are the basic steps: Stretch out on a carpeted floor in the basic relaxation pose. Do a brief scan of your body and release unnecessary muscular tension. Bring your right hand to rest over your

> **If you can consciously establish even, smooth, slow, diaphragmatic breathing, you will experience autonomic relaxation and be ready for sleep.**

navel and place your left hand on the middle of your chest. You will use your hands to monitor the motion of your abdomen and to make sure your chest remains still.

With your next exhalation, contract your abdominal muscles and feel the abdomen move down. Then relax your abdominal muscles; feel the inhalation coming into your lungs and feel your abdomen rising. Exhale again, contracting the abdomen. Inhale and relax the abdomen.

All of the motion associated with breathing should be centered in the abdomen. With your right hand you should feel the abdomen go down as you exhale and rise as you inhale. This is the most natural and efficient way to breathe. But when you first attend to your breath, it might feel strange or be hard to do. Just realize that as an infant or toddler you breathed diaphragmatically when you were content and happy. You are not learning something new, but relearning a way of breathing natural to you.

The exhalation is the active part of the breath. Consciously contract the abdominal muscles, pull them down and push the air out. With the inhalation just relax and let the air flow in. Keep working gently and patiently until this natural way of breathing comes back to you.

Once you establish the pattern of diaphragmatic breathing, try to make the inhalation and exhalation equal in length. Count the length of your exhalation and make the inhalation the same length. Work within your comfort-

All of the motion associated with breathing should be centered in the abdomen.

able capacity. You might begin with a count of three or four.

Next, make your breath smooth. Notice if you have a habit of pausing at the end of the inhalation or exhalation. Try to smooth it out so that your inhalation flows to a gradual end and then start with the beginning of your exhalation. Make an equally smooth transition from exhalation to inhalation. Watch your breath to see if you have any jerks or halts during the inhalation or exhalation. Smooth them out.

A ten- to twenty-minute session of diaphragmatic breathing can be a very useful relaxation exercise for your wind-down time. Such a session will reduce sympathetic activation and rebalance the ANS. It will clear your mind and calm your emotions. It will help you to shift from a vigilant, hyperalert state to a state of rest and relaxation.

Smooth, even diaphragmatic breathing can also be used as a key component of your sleep-time routine. Once you get into bed, practice diaphragmatic breathing. Slow your breathing and drift off to sleep naturally.

2:1 Breathing

As part of your sleep-time routine, you can also use a technique known as *2:1 breathing*. With this technique you make the exhalation twice as long as the inhalation. Because the exhalation enhances parasympathetic activation, 2:1 breathing induces a deep relaxation response and readily promotes the onset of sleep.

A ten- to twenty-minute session of diaphragmatic breathing can be a very useful relaxation exercise for your wind-down time.

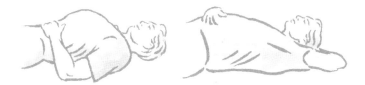

To practice this technique, exhale completely, counting the length of your exhalation. Inhale for half of that length. For most people this means starting with a count of six or eight on the exhalation and three or four on the inhalation. Remember to breathe diaphragmatically. Work within your comfortable capacity. As you gradually lengthen the exhalation and inhalation, you will have an effective means for creating autonomic relaxation and promoting the onset of complete, natural sleep.

The Brain and ANS Relaxation

The ANS is controlled by an area of the brain known as the *limbic system.* The limbic system is a thin layer of neural tissue situated between the brain stem and the cortex.

The limbic system selectively filters sensory data and orchestrates complex emotional responses. It is this system that analyzes what an animal smells, sees, and hears; perceives danger; and initiates a fight-or-flight response with strong emotions and strong autonomic activation.

There are several kinds of brain activity that influence

the limbic system and thereby the ANS. At the direct limbic level, this includes sensory information and emotions, while at the cortical level it includes images, words, and thoughts. We can manage these inputs to achieve ANS relaxation. Relaxation techniques based on these pathways include *autogenic training* and *visualization*.

Autogenic Training (AT)

Autogenic training is a method in which you create relaxation by thinking and inwardly repeating directives to relax specific body parts. The first step is *passive concentration.*

There are two key ingredients to achieving passive concentration. Select a comfortable and quiet environment and wear loose, easy-fitting clothes. Secondly, as you silently repeat an autogenic phrase, make mental contact with the part of the body you are addressing. For example, if the phrase is "My heartbeat is calm and regular," bring your full awareness to your heart. Generate a flow of visual, tactile, and auditory images to support the effect of the phrase. Hear the steady, comforting *babump* of the heartbeat, see the heart beating slowly and steadily, and feel it beating regularly in your chest. These words, images, and sensory experiences will influence the ANS. The images you choose should be pleasant and effective for you.

Autogenic relaxation is an effective technique for reducing sympathetic activation and calming the fight-or-flight

Autogenic training is a method in which you create relaxation by thinking and inwardly repeating directives to relax specific body parts.

response. The autogenic state is one of rest and relaxation and beautifully prepares you for sleep. Autogenic relaxation can be beneficially practiced as part of your wind-down routine, particularly if you are prone to autonomic tension. Once you have mastered autogenic relaxation, you can do an abbreviated session as part of your sleep-time routine.

THE PRACTICE OF AUTOGENIC RELAXATION

Stretch out in the basic relaxation pose. Utilize the techniques of passive concentration and silently repeat each autogenic phrase listed below three times. If it is comfortable, repeat the first half of the phrase as you inhale and the second half as you exhale. When you get to the heart, repeat that phrase and each subsequent phrase six times. Continue to focus your awareness on the body and generate a helpful stream of images and sensations. If you become distracted and lose your place, pick up wherever you think you left off.

At the end of the phrases, review the sensations throughout your body; breathe diaphragmatically and rest for a few moments. Then open your eyes, take a long stretch over your head, and roll to one side before you sit up.

Focus your awareness on the body and generate a helpful stream of images and sensations.

My right arm is heavy.

My left arm is heavy.

Both arms are heavy.

My right leg is heavy.

My left leg is heavy.

Both legs are heavy.

My arms and legs are heavy.

My right arm is warm.

My left arm is warm.

Both arms are warm.

My right leg is warm.

My left leg is warm.

Both legs are warm.

My forehead is cool.

My arms and legs are warm.

My right arm is heavy and warm.

My left arm is heavy and warm.

Both arms are heavy and warm.

My right leg is heavy and warm.

My left leg is heavy and warm.

Both legs are heavy and warm.

My arms and legs are heavy and warm.

My heartbeat is calm and regular.

My breathing is smooth and even.

My abdomen is warm.

VISUALIZATION AND AUTONOMIC RELAXATION

Visualization is another effective technique for autonomic relaxation. The key elements of visualization are *vivid imagery*, and *positive* and *pleasing* content. When all the senses are employed and the mind is absorbed in a beautiful scene, feelings of happiness and tranquility emerge. The images and positive feelings access the limbic system, reducing sympathetic tension and creating balance in the ANS.

Visualization is a relaxation technique that can be used during your wind-down routine. Once you have become

When all the senses are employed and the mind is absorbed in a beautiful scene, feelings of happiness and tranquility emerge.

A pleasant visualiza-
tion can help
transition you into a
wonderful night
of complete, natural
sleep.

proficient and can use it to quickly decrease ANS tension, you may find that it is an effective element in your sleep-time routine. A pleasant visualization can help transition you into a wonderful night of complete, natural sleep.

The Practice of Visualization

There are many visualization techniques to choose from. One of the most effective is "The Favorite Place," in which you picture a favorite place in nature or a fondly recalled home or room. It could be a beach, forest, or mountain setting you have visited, a composite of places you have known, or a place that you can imagine. It can be the home you grew up in or the home of a relative or grandparent. What's most important is that you can vividly recall the place and that it engenders positive feelings.

Select a quiet, comfortable room and stretch out in the basic relaxation pose or sit comfortably in a soft chair. Take several deep breaths and then establish even, smooth diaphragmatic breathing. Do a brief, guided relaxation to let go of any muscular tension.

In your mind begin to picture your favorite place. Experience a specific aspect of that place with one of your senses. Perhaps start by seeing the colors. If it is a beach, see the various blue or green hues of the water. If it is a room, recall the color of the walls or floor.

Then move to another specific sensory experience. Feel

the texture of the sand with your feet. Hear the sound of waves coming ashore. Smell the fresh sea air. If you are in a house, you can touch a familiar chair or inhale the aroma of your grandmother's freshly baked chocolate chip cookies.

After you have gone through all the senses once, then carefully go through them a second time. See the colors of the sky. Feel the temperature of the sand on your feet or feel the wind and warmth against your face. Hear the shorebirds calling or the sound of friendly, loving voices. Smell the pine needles or the scent of freshly washed clothes.

When you complete this second tour with your senses, take a third and fourth tour. Each time see, feel, hear, and smell another aspect of your favorite place. Fully immerse yourself in the experience. If you drift off, or the setting changes or evolves, that is fine. Just start in again with your in-depth sensory tours. Let the pleasant feelings of happiness, contentment, and harmony arise.

After ten to twenty minutes, gently bring your sensory awareness back to the present. Take several deep breaths, gently wiggle your fingers and toes to reactivate your muscles, and, when you are ready, open your eyes. Reach your arms over your head and take a long, lazy stretch. Roll to one side and get up when you are ready. This relaxation will help calm your autonomic nervous system, assist you in switching out of an alert, active, and vigilant mode, and prepare you for the nightly rest and regeneration you need.

This relaxation will prepare you for the nightly rest and regeneration you need.

sleep and
the
quiet mind

The mind is a field of intelligent energy in constant motion.
Like a crazed monkey jumping around in a tree, the mind
hops from one thing to another, often making unexpected
and undesirable leaps and turns.

Phil Nuernberger, *The Quest for Personal Power*

E ven when your muscles are relaxed and your nervous system balanced, mental tension may prevent you from falling asleep. As you lie quietly in bed, hoping to fall asleep, you notice that your mind is racing. Your mind re-creates the events of the day and reminds you of what you have to do tomorrow. You recall the upsetting things other people said and did. You replay your own responses and imagine what you could have said and done differently.

Your mind may bring up memories of past failures and achievements. You might anxiously rehearse for a challenging work assignment or nervously anticipate an exciting trip. You worry about money, relationships, family, health, and work. All this mental activity keeps you awake. And then you begin to worry if you will ever fall asleep.

All of this is the experience of mental tension. Even though your body is relaxed and your room is dark, you just can't stop the ceaseless activity of your mind. Mental tension can be a formidable barrier to sleep.

To remove this barrier, you need to understand the

Even though your body is relaxed and your room is dark, you just can't stop the ceaseless activity of your mind.

nature of the mind and to learn about the causes and types of mental tension. You need to understand the various ways that mental tension can disrupt sleep. And most importantly, you need to learn how to eliminate mental tension so you can enjoy complete, natural sleep.

THE NATURE OF THE MIND

The mind is that element or complex of elements in an individual that perceives, thinks, wills, and reasons. The mind is housed in the *cortex*, the large top part of the brain.

From the moment we wake up, our conscious mind constantly perceives sights, sounds, sensations, smells, and tastes. Perception is accompanied by inner talk. As we react, we might say to ourselves, "This room is chilly," "The lights are too bright," or "That coffee smells good."

We use this inner language when we plan, remember, problem solve, and worry. We talk to ourselves while we are driving, cooking, or playing. Sometimes the inner dialogue is accompanied by images in our mind's eye or sounds in our mind's ear. All this activity—this perception, this inner chatter, these images and sounds—runs through our mind ceaselessly throughout the day, creating mental tension. And when we can't turn it off at night, we just can't fall asleep.

From the moment we wake up, our conscious mind constantly perceives sights, sounds, sensations, smells, and tastes.

MENTAL TENSION

One of the most common forms of mental tension is the *scattered mind.* Here, our inner dialogue jumps from one subject to the next. We think about the past and we worry about the future. We think of things we would like to do and things we need to do. It is hard to concentrate on one thing because we are thinking about a thousand things. In terms of perception, we are likely to be hypervigilant. We hear and react to every sound; we see and react to every movement. Our attention flits from subject to subject.

With a scattered mind we feel at once wired yet tired. In terms of brain waves, the scattered mind is characterized by high-frequency beta waves from eighteen to twenty-two cps and a random rather than integrated pattern. The scattered mind tends to get more chaotic over time. The more we notice and react to, the more thoughts and ceaseless inner dialogue we generate.

Another type of tension is the *stuck mind.* Here, we get locked into a certain thought pattern, a repeating loop of inner dialogue, and we can't get away from it. We might find ourselves worrying about a job deadline, a relationship question, or an interpersonal conflict. We simply can't get the issue out of our mind. We keep replaying it again and again. We end up talking to ourselves in the same phrases and seeing the same images over and over and over.

> The more we notice and react to, the more thoughts and ceaseless inner dialogue we generate.

SLEEP AND THE QUIET MIND

The stuck mind is also very active and alert. But once again, behind the activity is often a sense of exhaustion. With the stuck mind, the brain waves will also stay in the high-frequency beta range but there may be actual hot spots where the brain is particularly active as it replays the same images and reruns the same words. For many people, mental tension is a combination of the scattered mind and the stuck mind.

Mental tension causes a qualitative shift in our consciousness. Our perception is narrowed and over-focused rather than open and flexible. We tend to lose any sense of being in the present and become preoccupied with the past and the future. We also get locked into the experience of binary consciousness, where we see differences and deficiencies. We are judgmental and critical. We experience isolation and separateness.

Mental tension also impairs the effectiveness of our thinking process. Our concentration is weaker. We are less able to focus deeply and problem solve. And we are less open and less creative.

Since the mind is the control room of the body and feelings, mental tension has a profound impact on our emotions, autonomic nervous system, and muscles. When our mind is scattered or stuck, we feel anxious, angry, and sad. These emotions activate the autonomic fight-or-flight response and cause us to tighten and brace our muscles.

When our mind is scattered or stuck, we feel anxious, angry, and sad.

The Impact of Mental Tension on Sleep

Mental tension interferes with falling asleep. Perhaps one of the most common complaints associated with insomnia is "I get into bed but I just can't shut off my mind." And this is understandable. The scattered or stuck mind is part of an activated alert state, the very opposite of a restful, ready-for-sleep state. When we go to bed with a tense mind, we are going to feel emotionally on edge, revved up within, and physically restless and tense.

Mental tension also interferes with staying asleep. If we wake up during the night, all the worries and thoughts are still racing through our mind, making it hard to fall back asleep. Mental tension is also associated with early wakening. It seems the tense mind breaks through our sleep and we wake up way too early.

In addition to these general effects, there are some very specific effects of mental tension. Amid the ceaseless inner chatter that makes up mental tension, there are often specific counterproductive self-talks that interfere with sleep.

People with sleep difficulties will often begin to worry about sleep during the day, telling themselves, "I'll probably have another bad night of sleep." When they get into bed, they think, "I'll never fall asleep." And when they have difficulty sleeping, they tell themselves, "If I don't get enough sleep, I just won't be able to function." And when they wake up after a bad night of sleep, they say, "After that night, I

> When we go to bed with a tense mind, we are going to feel emotionally on edge, revved up within, and physically restless and tense.

will never get through the day."

These thoughts could be called *Sleep-Ruining Thoughts*, or SRTs. They make us worried and agitated and make it even harder to fall asleep. Sometimes they become self-fulfilling prophesies. When we tell ourselves enough times that we can't sleep and that we will feel awful the next day, there is a pretty good chance these predictions will come true. SRTs make a bad situation worse.

A final effect of mental tension on sleep is something that could be called *sleep watching*. This occurs when we get into bed and then constantly watch and talk to ourselves about whether we are falling asleep. Sleep is run by unconscious centers in the brain. We don't need the activity of the conscious mind to help with sleep onset. In fact, watching, thinking, and worrying about falling asleep will just interfere with the process.

Eliminating Sleep-Ruining Thoughts

To eliminate harmful SRTs, we need to become aware of which ones are looping through our mind. Then we need to examine and challenge these SRTs. Most SRTs are not factually accurate. The beliefs we have about our sleep are often contrary to the facts of sleep science. Armed with accurate facts, we can refute these SRTs. And we can replace them with Sleep-Promoting Thoughts (SPTs). These SPTs can reduce our anxiety about sleep and help us to create

> When we tell ourselves enough times that we can't sleep and that we will feel awful the next day, there is a pretty good chance these predictions will come true.

positive and helpful expectations.

We will go through a number of common SRTs, proceeding more or less chronologically. In each case we will look at the negative impact of the thought, then use the facts of sleep science to refute the SRT, and, finally, replace the SRT with an SPT.

SRT #1: "I am sure I'll have a hard time falling asleep again tonight."

Impact: This thought can occur throughout the day, creating anxiety about sleep that builds up and interferes with falling asleep. It also creates a feeling of helplessness and a sense that you have no active control over your sleep.

Facts: It is natural to fall asleep at night. There are many things you can do during the course of the day to improve your sleep. These include reducing caffeine intake, being active, getting out in the sunlight, and implementing effective wind-down, bedtime, sleep-time, and wake-up routines. If you become active in choosing the right behaviors to improve your sleep, you will most likely enjoy better sleep. You are not helpless. You can make your sleep better.

SPT #1: "If I make the right choices and do the right things, I will get a good night's sleep."

SRT #2: "I'll never fall asleep."

Impact: This thought is surely one of the most damag-

You are not helpless. You can make your sleep better.

ing SRTs. It immediately increases your anxiety level, increases muscular tension, sets off an inner autonomic response, and creates an active and alert state that makes it harder to fall asleep. This SRT also leads you to watch your sleep, which further interferes with falling asleep.

Facts: Your brain and body are designed to fall asleep. At night your body temperature drops, melatonin levels rise, and sleep debt is present. All the natural ingredients are there to help you sleep. You can prepare yourself for sleep via your wind-down and bedtime routines. Once you are in bed, you can do muscular and autonomic relaxation techniques to help with sleep onset. And you can do mental relaxation and mental distraction techniques to help the natural process of sleep onset.

SPT #2: "It is natural to fall asleep, and I can do many things to help the process along."

SRT #3: "If I don't get enough sleep, I will never be able to function tomorrow."

Impact: This thought can occur when you get to bed late, are awakened during the night, or have to get up early. Like the others, this SRT will make you feel anxious and worried, set off the muscular and autonomic responses associated with anxiety, and make it harder to sleep.

Facts: Sleep is inherently resilient. There are two key dimensions to this resiliency. The first involves the concept

All the natural ingredients are there to help you sleep.

of *core sleep*. Remember, if you get about 5.5 hours of so-called core sleep, you will be able to function pretty well the next day. In fact, people can survive for several months on core sleep and suffer no ill consequences. The second dimension of resiliency has to do with the way your brain arranges for you to catch up on needed sleep. If you miss sleep tonight, you accumulate sleep debt and your brain will attempt to recover the amount and stage of sleep that you missed. In short, whatever you miss tonight you will recoup tomorrow night. And you can help the process by getting up at your regular time, maintaining your regular activity during the day, and following through with your normal wind-down and bedtime routines.

SPT #3: "Even if I miss some sleep tonight, I will be fine tomorrow and I will recoup the sleep I need tomorrow night."

SRT #4: "I'll never get back to sleep."

Impact: If you awaken during the night and have to attend to a crying child or a pet or to go to the bathroom, you may be somewhat alert when you get back into bed. If you have a little trouble falling asleep and begin to think this SRT, it will have the same effect as SRT #1. It will make you anxious, ignite muscular and autonomic tension, and make it all that much harder to fall back asleep.

Facts: It is quite common to wake up during the night.

> If you get about 5.5 hours of so-called core sleep, you will be able to function pretty well the next day.

And it is equally common to fall back asleep. You can use the same techniques of muscular relaxation, autonomic balance, and mental calming to fall back asleep. Most people fall back asleep in five to ten minutes.

SPT #4: "It is very common to wake up during the night and completely natural to fall back asleep after a few minutes. I can help the process along."

SRT #5: "After a terrible night's sleep like that, I am never going to be able to make it through the day."

Impact: This SRT makes a bad situation worse. After a night of restless or abbreviated sleep, this SRT sets up self-fulfilling negative expectations for the day. It is likely to make you feel discouraged, anxious, and even helpless as you face the day. In this frame of mind you are likely to engage in counterproductive behaviors such as consuming too much caffeine and giving up your normal activity-and-exercise routine.

Facts: In the morning, your body organizes for alertness and activity no matter what kind of sleep you received. Your body temperature rises, cortisol levels increase, and your morning surge of alertness takes over. One of the best things you can do is to carry out your normal routine. Get up at your regular time, do your morning stretches or exercise, take a refreshing morning shower, and get a good breakfast. You will be just fine during the day. Keep yourself active.

In the morning, your body organizes for alertness and activity no matter what kind of sleep you received.

Maintain your wind-down and bedtime routines and you will recoup any lost sleep the next night. If you feel a little more tired than usual during your afternoon dip, you can do a few stretches or take a relaxation break.

SPT #5: "Even if I didn't sleep that great, I will be just fine during the day and I can do a lot of things to get myself back on track for a good night's sleep tonight."

These are five of the most common and destructive SRTs. You may have some of these or a few unique variations. Whatever your personal SRTs are, it is important to identify them and revise them. It may be helpful for you to write down your SRTs and then write a replacement SPT. It is crucial that you learn to catch yourself in the act. At that moment during the day or night when you think an SRT, you need to catch it, challenge it, and rephrase it.

Initially, this may be difficult because your SRTs have become automatic and habitual. But gradually you can break the SRT habit and through your direct experience realize that the SPTs are both true and helpful. Your new SPTs will put you back in charge of your sleep and help you to obtain complete, natural sleep.

MENTAL RELAXATION

Now that we have dealt with specific thoughts that interfere

At that moment when you think an SRT, you need to catch it, challenge it, and rephrase it.

with sleep, we are ready to learn about overall mental relaxation. Remember, a tense mind is both scattered and stuck and characterized by rapid and random brain waves. A tense mind is locked into an alert, activated, hypervigilant state that makes it hard to fall asleep.

A relaxed mind is *focused*. As the mind becomes absorbed in one topic, it stops jumping from thought to thought and worry to worry. We all know how relaxing it can be when we are totally involved in a book or a craft project. For a little while we forget about everything else as we focus deeply on one thing. After an interval of such deep focus, we often feel refreshed and renewed.

Openness is another quality of the relaxed mind. Instead of being reactive and judgmental, we become fully open and aware. We notice more but react less. We become conscious of the sounds and sights in the environment, of the people around us, and of our own experience. But our awareness is open, flowing, and nonjudgmental.

The relaxed mind also tends to be *present centered*. Instead of thinking about the past and the future, we are fully responsive to the present moment. Worries about yesterday and tomorrow fade as we experience the richness of the present moment. As a result, we begin to experience a more unitary consciousness.

The relaxed mind is also characterized by *changes in the brain waves*. The brain slows down to the alpha

The relaxed mind also tends to be present centered. Instead of thinking about the past and the future, we are fully responsive to the present moment.

range of eight to twelve cps. The brain waves are integrated and harmonious.

A relaxed mind is open to the natural onset of sleep. And when we fall asleep with a relaxed mind, we are likely to sleep soundly straight through the night and awaken refreshed and renewed. Now let us learn several methods of mental relaxation.

CONCENTRATION

One method of mental relaxation is known as *concentration*. This method uses the principles of focus and present-centered awareness to create mental relaxation. During the practice of concentration, the mind is focused on one thing rather than jumping from one subject to the next. Just as a scattered and distracted mind indicates tension, a centered and focused mind is a sign of relaxation.

When your mind has a firmly established habit of jumping from one topic to the next, it may take some effort to change that pattern and to focus on one thing. But when you can consciously sustain true concentration, you will begin to achieve deep mental relaxation.

The following concentration technique uses breath as a point of focus. You can either read through and memorize these instructions or tape-record them.

A centered and focused mind is a sign of relaxation.

The Practice of Concentration

In a quiet room, sit toward the front edge of a firm chair. Bend your knees so that your feet rest flat on the floor. Bring your shoulders back and bring a natural curve into your lower back. Align your head so that your ears are above your shoulders and your lower back.

Bring your full awareness to your breath.

Close your eyes. Take several deep breaths. Then settle into even, smooth, diaphragmatic breathing. Do a brief guided relaxation. Let go of tension throughout your body.

Bring your full awareness to your breath. Breathe diaphragmatically. Your abdomen moves in with the exhalation and out with the inhalation. Your chest is still. Make sure your breath is even and smooth.

Focus your awareness on your breath as it flows in and out of your nose. As the air flows in, it feels cool and dry. As the air flows out, it feels warm and moist.

Don't evaluate or react. Just keep your focus on the even, smooth, diaphragmatic breathing and the sensation of cool, dry air flowing in and warm, moist air flowing out. If you get distracted or drift off, that is very natural. Just bring your awareness back to your breath.

Keep the experience easy and comfortable. Check the muscles in your face for any tension and relax them. Continue to focus on the breath—cool, dry air in and warm, moist air flowing out.

Maintain your focus on the breath for a comfortable

interval of time. At the beginning, this may be five to ten minutes. With practice, you will be able to concentrate up to twenty minutes.

When you are done, gently open your eyes. Let your breathing become more active, and take a nice, long stretch.

This concentration technique can be done as part of your wind-down routine to help you relax and clear your mind. Concentration can be a beneficial part of your wake-up routine as well, helping you start the day with a clear and focused mind. Concentration can also be very helpful during your midafternoon lull to give you conscious rest.

MEDITATION

An even deeper level of mental relaxation can be achieved through the practice of *meditation.* Many people think that meditation means thinking deeply or pondering a subject. But really it is a way to work with the mind, not a type of thinking. Meditation is a conscious process of focusing the mind in a nonanalytic manner.

Meditation is the unbroken flow of thought toward an object of concentration. The object might be a word, an image, a picture, or a concept. If the object is a specific word, start with concentration. As your concentration deepens, your mind flows continuously toward the word. As you move deeper into meditation, your mind becomes

Meditation is a conscious process of focusing the mind in a nonanalytic manner.

totally absorbed in the word.

Meditation creates a profound state of mental relaxation characterized by slow, regular, and integrated brain waves. During meditation the thinking process is stilled and the mind becomes quiet. The meditator is fully in the present, feels peace and contentment, and experiences a sense of unitary consciousness.

Meditation seems to have a number of beneficial effects on sleep. People who practice meditation daily seem to have an easier time letting go of worries and concerns and drifting off to sleep.

Regular meditators seem to need less sleep. This may be due to an overall healthier lifestyle. It may be due to getting a little extra sleep by dozing off during meditation. Or it may be that by consciously slowing the mind, they fulfill a part of their sleep need. Whatever the reason, meditation is the finest form of mental relaxation.

Meditation can be done as part of your wind-down routine or you can practice in the morning as part of your wake-up routine. Starting the day with meditation is one way to keep the mind more relaxed throughout the day.

The Practice of Meditation

The accompanying CD includes a guided meditation. Here are some additional guidelines:

Set aside a regular time for meditation. That way you

The meditator is fully in the present, feels peace and contentment, and experiences a sense of unitary consciousness.

don't have to decide each day when you are going to meditate, but will have a positive habit. Early in the morning, at midday, late afternoon, or in the evening before bed are all good times. Start off by meditating for five to ten minutes and gradually work up to twenty to thirty minutes.

Set aside a specific place to meditate. Choose a spot that is quiet and pleasant and has a flow of fresh air. As time goes by you will develop an association to this spot and it will feel natural to sit there and meditate.

A number of steps can help you prepare for meditation. These should be seen as guidelines but not fixed rules. Prepare for meditation by taking a shower or washing your face and hands. Avoid eating for a few hours before you meditate. Wear loose, comfortable but warm clothing. Do a few stretches to get rid of muscular tension.

Assume a firm but comfortable posture. Your back should be naturally curved, your shoulders, back, and head aligned. You can sit on the front edge of a chair with your feet on the floor. You can sit on the front edge of a firm cushion on the floor with your legs crossed. Or if you are flexible, you can sit on the floor, bend your right leg, and place the sole of your right foot against your left thigh. Bring your left ankle under your right ankle and position the sole of your left foot against your right

Start off by meditating for five to ten minutes and gradually work up to twenty to thirty minutes.

thigh. Place a firm cushion under your buttocks to increase your comfort and to create a natural curve in your lower back.

Select an object of meditation. Counting each exhalation, starting at one and going up to ten and beginning again, is a traditional Zen practice that is good for beginning meditators. A *mantra* is a specific word designed to be an object of meditation. A traditional yogic mantra pairs the sound *so* with the inhalation and the sound *hum* with the exhalation. *So* means "that" and *hum* means "I am." Put together, the phrase means "that I am" or "that inner spiritual self is my real self."

As you did with concentration, start by closing your eyes, breathing diaphragmatically, and doing a brief guided relaxation to let go of any muscular tension. Then begin to focus your mind on the object of meditation you have selected. Little by little, become absorbed in the object of meditation. Don't struggle. If you lose track, just start over. If thoughts, emotions, or memories come up, notice them and then let go. If you get distracted by sounds, notice them, let go, and bring your mind back to the object of meditation. If your body becomes uncomfortable, just notice that, let go, and return your awareness to the object of meditation. Even if creative thoughts and exciting plans emerge, just notice them and let go. After you have dealt with any of these distractions, return to smooth diaphrag-

Counting each exhalation is a traditional Zen practice that is good for beginning meditators.

matic breathing, restore your balanced and firm posture, and bring your focus back to the object of meditation.

When you have finished your allotted time, take several deep breaths, gently open your eyes, and take a nice, long stretch. Sit and reflect for a few minutes or get up and resume your activities. After a session of meditation, your mind will be relaxed, rested, and refreshed.

After a session of meditation your mind will be relaxed, rested, and refreshed.

OVERCOMING SLEEP WATCHING

The final type of mental tension we need to address is the very counterproductive habit of watching the process of falling asleep. If you lie in bed and focus on whether or not you are falling asleep, you will definitely prevent sleep onset.

The traditional technique of counting sheep is a way to get the mind off falling asleep. You busy your mind counting sheep, and before you know it, you have fallen asleep. There are actually more effective techniques to occupy the mind and distract its thoughts from the process of falling asleep.

To begin, you want to select something that is pleasant and mildly compelling to think about. For example, people who are golfers can pick a favorite course, picture it vividly, and imagine playing each hole shot by shot. You can recall a favorite house or building and take a tour through each room and floor. You can recall a favorite hike and see yourself passing familiar landmarks as you travel down the path. Or perhaps you can recall a pleasant musical composition or movie.

You can also simply recall all the details of your day, starting with your morning routine and then following through the events of the day. Remember such details as what was on the radio or TV as you dressed, what you had for breakfast, and so on. Try to imagine you are watching a movie of your day. Chances are that as you recall today, before you know it, you will fall asleep and the next thing you know, tomorrow will have arrived.

The best themes have a pleasant association. Ideally, the theme will have some type of progression to keep your conscious mind moving while your unconscious mind orchestrates your passage into sleep. Any of the approaches described above, or others you invent, will help eliminate sleep watching and allow you to fall asleep naturally.

Another good technique for engaging the conscious mind is to practice a systematic relaxation technique. For example, you can do a guided relaxation starting at your feet and working your way up to your forehead. You can also practice 2:1 breathing with the exhalation twice as long as the inhalation. These help distract the conscious mind and relax the body, a perfect combination to help you fall asleep.

Try to imagine you are watching a movie of your day.

spiritual
resources to
improve
sleep

A clear conscience is the best pillow.

Anonymous

E ven when your mind is quiet, your nervous system balanced, and your muscles relaxed, you may notice a tension deep within that disturbs your sleep. This tension may include feelings of discontent, loneliness, even guilt. You may feel conflict about priorities in your life. You might question the purpose and meaning of your life. You may worry if you are doing the right kind of work or living in the right place.

You may notice that you don't look forward to getting up in the morning nor do you have a sense of peace when you go to bed at night. You may even notice that you have fears about your own death.

These are the signs of spiritual tension, a subtle yet pervasive tension that corrodes the quality of our life and undermines the quality of our sleep. To attain the best sleep, we need to learn to ease this spiritual tension.

THE SPIRITUAL LEVEL

The spiritual level is at once the most compelling plane of human existence and the most challenging to describe and define. While spiritual concerns are a central part of our life,

The spiritual level is at once the most compelling plane of human existence and the most challenging to define.

One of the most
universal themes is
a belief in an aspect
of life that lies
beyond the ordinary,
beyond that which
can be weighed and
measured—a sacred
dimension.

there is no clear-cut physiological system where our spiritual sensibilities reside. Yet in our hearts and minds we feel and know the spiritual dimension of life is real and important.

We can define this level by looking at some of the persistent themes that run through our spiritual life. One of the most universal of these is a belief in an aspect of life that lies beyond the ordinary, beyond that which can be weighed and measured—a sacred dimension. Most cultures throughout history have found both peace and order in life through acknowledging a power beyond human capability. Reverence for this higher power has been an essential aspect of the spiritual nature of humankind.

This sacred dimension has been viewed as imbued with qualities that influence and direct daily life. Ancient cultures believed these spiritual forces resided in those aspects of nature that sustained life. As a result, they worshipped the sun, the moon, and the fertility of plants and humans.

In ancient Greek and Roman religion, the sacred dimension contained an array of gods and goddesses who managed nature and presided over war, love, science, and wisdom. Worship of a particular god or goddess via sacrifice or prayer was designed to bring a specific aspect of the sacred dimension into one's life.

In monotheistic religions, spiritual power resides in a single ultimate being who is viewed as transcendent yet involved in human affairs.

SPIRITUAL TENSION

Spiritual tension occurs when we lack a meaningful relationship to the sacred. As a result, we are likely to feel isolated and disconnected. There is little to look forward to and life becomes a matter of putting in time.

Spiritual tension often leads to cynicism. In the absence of a spiritual perspective, we come to believe that immediate self-interest is the only motivating force in people. Consequently, we become disillusioned in civic, social, and religious institutions. Without a relationship to the sacred, we lose a sense of purpose and direction in life.

In the absence of a spiritual perspective, we may not have an ethical or behavioral code to support our personal conscience. We may subscribe to the philosophy that there is no real right or wrong. As a result, we may drift through life like a rudderless boat, feeling conflicted about what we have done and what we have failed to do.

When there is spiritual tension, we are cut off from guidance from a higher level. We lack spiritual input to help us make difficult decisions, to guide us through tough times, to help us chart the best path of personal development. When there is spiritual tension, we feel inner restlessness, a lack of inner peace. We find it difficult to be content with our place in the world.

Without a relationship to the sacred, we lose a sense of purpose and direction in life.

THE EFFECT OF SPIRITUAL TENSION ON SLEEP

When we go to bed with spiritual tension, we are likely to feel a sense of uneasiness. One part of this uneasiness may be a lack of contentment and satisfaction. Or the uneasiness may be made up of questioning and conflict about how our life is going.

This uneasiness then creates tension on the mental level. We may think and worry about our direction in life, about the meaning and satisfaction inherent in what we have done during the day. This mental tension is quickly translated into rapid brain waves, autonomic activation, and muscular tension. And soon we are agitated, restless, and can't fall asleep.

This uneasiness may lead to emotional tension. We may be gripped by anxiety about the future, guilt about the past, anger about mistreatment by others, frustration that we are denied what we desire, disgust with our inadequacies, and fears about illness and death. Wracked by these negative emotions, we find it difficult to fall asleep.

Sometimes with spiritual tension we lack motivation to establish and stick to a healthy sleep routine. If everything is relative and nothing matters, then why go to bed at a regular time? If there is no imperative to respect and care for our bodies as extensions of the sacred, then it doesn't matter when and how we sleep.

When we go to bed with spiritual tension, we are likely to feel a sense of uneasiness.

Given the many negative effects of spiritual tension and its impact on sleep, let us now explore those spiritual perspectives and practices that can help us sleep better.

THE SABBATH PERSPECTIVE

One of the biggest problems affecting sleep is that we simply don't value it. We don't view sleep as a positive, creative aspect of life, but as something that encroaches on time that could better be spent in some profitable external activities. When we embrace this view of sleep as a necessary evil, a biologically mandated waste of time, then we look for ways to cut corners on sleep.

But if we look within the spiritual traditions, we find the notion of Sabbath, a time set aside for rest, a time of quiet and peace, a time dedicated to the life within, a time for connection with the sacred. Perhaps this notion of Sabbath can help us to view rest in general and sleep in particular as both needed antidotes to the hectic pace of modern life and as positive and creative forces in life.

The word *Sabbath* comes from the Hebrew *Shabbath*, which means "rest." In Judaism, the Sabbath is a Biblically mandated day of rest that is a central element of spiritual life. The mandate is found in the book of Genesis, where God blessed the seventh day and rested after his mighty task of creation, and in Exodus, where the people of Israel are

One of the biggest problems affecting sleep is that we simply don't value it.

commanded to work six days but to keep the seventh free of work—as a day of rest.

But the Sabbath is more than just a day of the week. It is a revolutionary concept that introduces the sacred into the way we use time. The notion of Sabbath provides a spiritual directive to set aside time for rest.

Within the notion of Sabbath, rest is not passive. It is not just a day off, but a creative force. Sabbath is a balance. It is a time of dormancy to be followed by a rebirth. It is a time of stillness that draws on healing forces from within and restores our life energy.

We can apply the notion of Sabbath to our daily routine. We can dedicate time for sleep. We can come to regard sleep as a dynamic, creative, and healing force. We can appreciate sleep as a necessary balance in our life. Every day we can enjoy the blessing of sleep and restore our mind, body, and spirit.

SPIRITUAL PRACTICES THROUGH THE DAY

Many of the great religions of the world view the passage of each day as a sacred cycle, as a direct opportunity to interact with the sacred. Accordingly, there are spiritual practices of prayer and worship linked to specific times of day. Many of these practices frame the hours of sleep.

The morning is an opportunity for starting the day

with a sense of spiritual attunement and purpose. The evening allows us to process the experiences of the day and to enter into the realm of sleep with a sense of peace. Within the religious traditions of the world, we can find prayers for the morning and evening that we can bring into our daily sleep routine.

THE NATURE OF PRAYER

The word "pray" comes from the Latin word "to ask." When we ask during prayer, we are entering into communication and relationship with the sacred. Prayers should be given with single-minded attention, free of expectation and ego. Prayers should be spoken with belief and sincerity.

Prayer is inner speech. We say and think the prayer within. Or we can say the prayer aloud. Sometimes we may hold an image in our mind as we pray. Prayer can be practiced standing, sitting, walking, or kneeling. A standing position implies honor and respect, while bending the head forward brings a sense of humility. Closing the eyes during prayer can help us to focus and bring our attention within.

Prayer can be one of the most effective means for reducing spiritual tension in our life. Prayer can offer solace and support when we are down. Through prayer we can express gratitude and thanks for the many blessings in our life. And prayer can be an avenue for receiving guidance and

Prayers should be spoken with belief and sincerity.

finding meaning and purpose in life.

EVENING PRAYERS

In the evening our body quiets down. The business of the day is completed. The evening is a time to prepare ourselves for sleep. Through prayer we can let go of the worries of the day, establish a sense of peace, and seek comfort and protection for our journey through the night.

The Benefits of Evening Prayer

Evening prayer themes can assist in eliminating spiritual tension that interferes with sleep. One helpful theme in evening prayers is *forgiveness*. We ask forgiveness for our mistakes in word, deed, and thought. Forgiveness can ease our guilt and lessen our self-condemnation. It allows us to let go of the mistakes of the day and to sleep peacefully. And as we sense forgiveness for ourselves, we are able to offer it to others and let go of our anger.

Another theme is *protection*. As we begin the journey into the dark night, into the unknown realm of sleep, we ask for protection. We petition the sacred to watch over us and our loved ones and to keep us safe through the night. With this protection we feel comfort. Our anxieties and fears are diminished.

Associated with protection is the idea of *surrender*. We

take ourselves off duty and trust God to stay on duty to protect us. A burden is lifted from our shoulders. We can relax.

Thanksgiving is a part of many evening prayers. Before
we fall asleep we express our gratitude for all the blessings
we have received during the day. We give thanks for the
material benefits of the day, the food, shelter, and clothing.
We offer gratitude for the friends and loved ones who are in
our life. These expressions of thanksgiving bring feelings of
happiness and contentment, of gratitude and fulfillment.

Peace is another theme in evening prayers. After the
struggles of the day, we ask for peace. This peace can soothe
our mind, balance our nervous system, relax our muscles,
and prepare the way for sleep.

Evening prayers also ask for *complete rest* so that we can
enjoy the full purpose of sleep and be refreshed and renewed
for the next day, so that we can awaken the next morning
energized to follow our vocation and achieve our purpose in
life.

Sleep is also an opportunity for guidance. After a good
night's sleep, we can awaken with a clear vision of what we
need to do, of the right course of action. And during the
hours of sleep, we may receive dreams that will give us guidance and answer our questions.

Evening prayers can be offered during your wind-down
time. You can make up your own prayers. You can explore
your own religious traditions to find prayers that ease your

Expressions of thanksgiving bring feelings of happiness and contentment, of gratitude and fulfillment.

spiritual tension.

Evening prayers can even be part of your sleep-time routine. When you fill your mind and heart with a prayer as you slip into bed, you will banish negative thoughts and emotions. As you repeat the prayer, you not only avoid sleep watching, but you create positive and beneficial thoughts and feelings to carry you into sleep.

MORNING PRAYERS

Morning is another beneficial time for prayer. During the freshness of the morning and before we become preoccupied with the activities of the day, we can be particularly open to the effect of prayer. Just as a breath of fresh air, morning sunlight, and a nice stretch can awaken the body and senses, prayer can awaken the mind and heart. Prayer can help us set a tone for the day. Morning prayer can bring meaning and purpose into our day. Getting spiritually attuned to start the day makes it worthwhile to get up and worthwhile to sleep well.

The Benefits of Morning Prayer

Morning prayers share many themes with evening prayers: protection, peace, compassion, patience, and expressions of thanksgiving for a night of peaceful rest and a day of fresh opportunities. Morning prayers can contribute to an

Morning prayer can bring meaning and purpose into our day.

enthusiastic and optimistic outlook. Morning prayers can also help us overcome any feelings of fear and anxiety about the day ahead.

Perhaps one of the most consistent themes in morning prayers is guidance—guidance in our dealings with others and in dealing with the ups and downs of the day, and guidance in finding purpose and meaning in life. Morning prayer can restore our hope and enthusiasm.

SLEEP AND THE SPECTRUM OF SPIRITUAL PRACTICES

While prayer can directly frame going to sleep and rising, there are many other spiritual practices that can support the broader themes of bringing meaning and purpose to our lives.

Weekly worship, regular study of scriptures, fellowship, singing of hymns and sacred music, and acts of community service and charity are all beneficial forms of spiritual practice. Research tells us that people who have these elements of spiritual practice in their life and who see the sacred as benevolent and loving cope better with stress. They are simply more resilient during the tough times. They experience less depression and anxiety. Their physical health is better.

People whose lives include spiritual practice also sleep better. There are probably many reasons for this. One may

Weekly worship, regular study of scriptures, fellowship, singing of hymns and sacred music, and acts of community service and charity are all beneficial forms of spiritual practice.

be having a more regular schedule. Another may stem from having more frequent feelings of forgiveness, peace, support, and protection. And yet another may be the ability to turn over one's cares at night to let go of struggling, to enter tranquilly the realm of sleep where body, mind, and spirit are restored.

overcoming sleep challenges: shift work, jet lag, and more

Ah, what is more blessed than to put cares away,
when the mind lays by its burden, and tired with
labor of far travel we have come to our own home
and rest on the couch we have longed for?

Catullus, 87-54 B.C.

T he ideal situation is one in which we can set up a regular sleep schedule that coincides with the natural rhythm of day and night. But all too often there are factors that interfere with our desire to live by this natural pattern.

These challenges include such modern phenomena as shift work and jet lag. Or we may find that our sleep is disrupted and curtailed because we are taking care of young children or a disabled or elderly parent or relative. We may find ourselves confronted with a crisis at work or have to cope with a natural disaster.

Sleep challenges such as these are common. They tax the natural resiliency of sleep. To cope with these sleep challenges, we need an effective approach.

THE PROBLEM OF SHIFT WORK

For thousands of years humankind has worked during the daylight hours and rested at night. With the advent of

We may find that our sleep is disrupted and curtailed because we are taking care of young children or a disabled or elderly parent or relative.

Women shift workers are more vulnerable to reproductive problems, including disrupted menstruation, more difficulty conceiving, more miscarriages, and more premature births.

electric lights it became possible to work through the night hours. With the new global twenty-four-hours-a-day economy, the use of shift work has increased dramatically. As a result, it is now estimated that 15 to 20 percent of the workforce is engaged in shift work.

Unfortunately, shift work has a number of negative effects. People are working when their bodies are tired and sleeping when their bodies want to be awake. Not surprisingly, anywhere from 50 to 80 percent of shift workers have sleep difficulties. These include trouble falling asleep and staying asleep. Shift workers are typically sleep deprived, as they receive about two hours less sleep per twenty-four-hour day than day workers. One effect of this sleep deprivation is falling asleep on the job. As many as two-thirds of shift workers fall asleep on the job at least once a week.

Shift work has other negative effects on health, including a higher incidence of gastrointestinal (GI) problems such as heartburn, diarrhea, constipation, and ulcers. Shift work raises the risk of cardiovascular disease by 30 to 50 percent. Women shift workers are more vulnerable to reproductive problems, including disrupted menstruation, more difficulty conceiving, more miscarriages, and more premature births.

Shift workers often experience decreased memory and concentration, as well as increased depression and anxiety. Shift workers may come to rely on caffeine, alcohol, and sleeping pills to cope with their schedule. They report decreased job satisfaction. Shift work also creates significant social stress. Married shift workers have less time with their spouse and children.

There are several types of shifts, some more stressful than others. Evening shifts that run from about 3 to 11 P.M. are easier to tolerate. Night shifts from about 11 P.M. until 7 A.M. are the most difficult, as they demand work during the early morning period when the body hits its daily low in activation and alertness. Clockwise rotating shifts change from days to evenings to nights and are generally easier to handle than counterclockwise shifts that go from days to nights to evenings. It may take between ten and fourteen days to adjust to a new shift schedule. Shifts that rotate more frequently than that are likely to be much more stressful.

Only 25 percent of shift workers actually choose to work at night. The other 75 percent work shifts because they have to. Some people never adjust to shift work, while others adjust with varying degrees of ease. Those who do adjust are typically under forty, in good health, and have a strong dedication to their work.

Coping with shift work demands a clear understanding of the importance of making an optimal adjustment. You can't just stick with your old daily routine and somehow get by. You need to organize your life and your sleep schedule

Coping with shift work demands a clear understanding of the importance of making an optimal adjustment.

Once you have
established a
routine, stick with
it as consistently
as possible.

around your shift work. Then will you be able to get the sleep you need to protect your health.

Coping with Shift Work

Many shift workers try to live in two worlds: that of their shift and that of the normal day schedule. As a result they sleep at different times on different days and try to be alert and active at different times. They end up not getting enough sleep and feeling completely out of sync with any type of schedule.

Perhaps the most important part of coping with shift work is to design a sleep schedule that allows you to get the sleep you need. It is crucial that you carve out a regular time for adequate sleep and stick with it. For example, if you get off work at 7 A.M., you may want to wind down for a while and then set aside from 8 A.M. to 3 P.M. to sleep. If you work an evening shift and get off work at midnight, again you can take some time to wind down and then go to sleep at 1 A.M. and rise at 9 A.M.

Once you have established a routine, stick with it as consistently as possible. Even on your days off, stay with your schedule. If you work the night shift, then on weekends you should stay up later and sleep later. On the weekends, you can budget extra time for sleep to ease any sleep debt that has accumulated during the work week.

Once you have a schedule, then create a complete sleep-promoting routine employing many of the techniques described in earlier chapters. Don't try to just jump into bed and fall asleep after your shift. Budget enough time to go through a wind-down routine, even if it is abbreviated.

Set up a regular bedtime routine. And follow through with your sleep-time routine of relaxation, visualization, mental distracters, and prayer. And when you get up, create a pleasant wake-up routine with stretches, washup, and exercise.

You will also need to do everything possible to ensure that you can sleep well during the day. First of all, make sure your room is completely dark. Use blackout shades or eyeshades. Secondly, control noise. Make sure your sleeping room is in a quiet part of your home. Use an air conditioner, a white-noise generator, or earplugs. Turn off the ringer on your phone and have calls go immediately into an answering machine. Keep the temperature cool in your bedroom.

You will need to be consistent and even strict about your sleeping routine. Make sure all your family members understand the importance of your sleep schedule. You can reassure them that by letting you sleep during the allotted time, they will help you to have more energy and time for them when you are awake. Let your neighbors and relatives know you do not want to be disturbed during your sleep time.

Make sure all your family members understand the importance of your sleep schedule.

A Sleep-Promoting Routine

During your waking hours, maintain a healthy sleep-promoting routine. Get adequate exercise. Eat healthy, nourishing food. Schedule social and recreational time. Often the inherent difficulties of shift work are compounded by poor lifestyle choices of fast food, excessive caffeine, increased alcohol consumption, and a sedentary lifestyle. If you are doing shift work it is even more important that you have a healthy, sleep-promoting lifestyle.

Plan your meals carefully. Avoid eating a big, heavy meal before you go to sleep or before you go to work. Schedule your biggest meal for sometime after you wake up. You may find it helpful to eat several smaller, lighter, and healthier meals throughout the day.

Use caffeine wisely to support a good sleep schedule. A cup of coffee to start your shift can be helpful. If you are working the night shift, it is normal for people to feel sleepiest at about 3 A.M. Drinking a cup of coffee or tea at 2:30 A.M. could help you get through this normally sleepy period. But don't rely on cup after cup of coffee to get you through the night when you are not getting the sleep you need during the day. And don't drink coffee during the four to six hours before you expect to go to sleep.

Use light to help you adjust to shift work. Exposure to light helps to make you alert and to reset your inner clock. If you work a night shift, avoid or minimize exposure to early morning sunlight, as this will make you feel more alert and will set your inner clock to an earlier schedule. Wear dark glasses on the way home. Once you get home, keep the lights low.

On the other hand, exposure to sunlight in the late afternoon or evening can help you feel alert and can help set your inner clock to a later schedule.

Look carefully at your work schedule. You may want to schedule the most challenging tasks early in your shift. Later in the shift you may want to look for opportunities to move around and perform tasks that help you stay alert. Exercise makes you feel more awake and attentive. You may want to schedule a brief break during your shift to do some stretches or take a walk.

Some people find that they can split up their sleep schedule and do quite well. For example, if they work the night shift, they can sleep for four or five hours in the morning, wake up and be active, and then sleep for another sixty to ninety minutes at night before they go to work. This way they are well rested when they get to work.

Look carefully at your work schedule. You may want to schedule the most challenging tasks early in your shift.

Naps and Shift Work

Some people find that even a short nap of twenty to thirty minutes before they go to work can be quite helpful. Most shift workers would benefit tremendously from being able to take a brief nap during their work time. Studies of long-haul airline pilots who were allowed to take a twenty-minute nap while the copilot had the controls showed that these pilots subsequently performed better and were much less likely to experience dangerous micro sleeps.

Naps as an aspect of sleep are not well understood. It is not clear exactly what happens in terms of sleep stages during naps. Nor is there any consensus on the optimal length of naps. For example, some people like a nap of thirty to sixty minutes while others feel better after a very brief nap of three to ten minutes. What research does consistently indicate is that subjects who have had even a brief nap show definite improvements in concentration, reaction time, alertness, and decision making.

These objective findings are often in conflict with what people feel subjectively. Some people report a kind of postnap inertia and grogginess. But surprisingly, in spite of these feelings, subjects still show improved functioning.

People who are experienced with relaxation may find it easy to rest when the opportunity presents itself. People who are skilled at relaxation can consciously create a state of deep relaxation that provides some of the benefits of a brief nap. Such conscious sleep may also be a useful tool in coping with the challenge of shift work.

Individual Sleep Patterns and Shift Work
Much of what has been listed above are general guidelines

Subjects who have had even a brief nap show definite improvements in concentration, reaction time, alertness, and decision making.

for dealing with shift work. But individuals vary considerably in how they respond and adjust to shift work. Some people adjust easily while others never adjust. For example, "owls" seem to have a much easier time adjusting to night work than do "larks." Individuals who biologically get by on six or seven hours of sleep may adjust better than those who require eight or nine hours of sleep.

Some people are simply more flexible and adaptable with their sleep. They can fall asleep anywhere and anytime, while others have to stick to a regular sleep routine. Some individuals can readily split up their sleep and take naps whenever the opportunity presents, while others can't. Knowing your unique sleep needs and sleep personality can help you cope with shift work.

JET LAG

In 1271 when Marco Polo made his epic trip from Europe to China, it took him three and a half years to arrive in Xanadu, the summer capital of the Mongol emperor Kublai Khan. As he journeyed eastward, his biological clock made the adjustment quite easily as he went along. When he reached China, he had traversed seven time zones and was none the worse for it.

But consider Marco's descendant, Giovanni. This modern man climbs aboard a jet in Venice at 5 P.M. and seven

> Individuals vary considerably in how they respond and adjust to shift work. Some people adjust easily while others never adjust.

hours later strides into the Beijing airport. Local time is 7 A.M., yet Giovanni's body tells him it is midnight.

Even though he is a little sleepy, he gets a cab to his hotel, checks in, unpacks, has a shower, and drinks a cup of tea to get ready for the day's events. At 10 A.M. when he is in an important meeting with a group of Chinese business-men, his body, set at Venice time, thinks it is 3 A.M. Body temperature and alertness are at their daily low. While his Chinese counterparts are discussing the fine details of a contract, poor Giovanni is fighting off sleep, can't concentrate, and can't remember important information.

Two hours later when his guests treat him to a sumptu-ous lunch, his body thinks it is 5 A.M. and he can hardly eat or digest the food. By midafternoon Giovanni might start to feel a little better as his body now thinks it is 8 A.M. At midnight Beijing time when he should be drifting off to sleep, his body thinks it is 5 P.M. Even though he has a huge sleep debt, he can't fall asleep. His body is ramping up for its second phase of alertness.

A week later, just as Giovanni is starting to adjust to Beijing time, he flies back to his home in Venice, only to discover that he is once again out of sync with his environment. Now he is ahead of local time.

During his time in China and after his return home, Giovanni has suffered from jet lag. His biological clock was out of sync with local time. His sleep cycle was thrown completely off. He had a hard time falling asleep, staying asleep, and getting the deep sleep that he needed.

The Effects of Jet Lag

Along with sleep disruption, he is likely to experience a number of other symptoms. He will notice that he feels tired and fatigued. He may have difficulty concentrating, remembering, and thinking. His sense of time will be off. He will process information more slowly. He is likely to suffer from digestive problems, including diarrhea and constipation. He might have headaches. He is likely to feel irritable, short-tempered, and out of sorts.

Millions of people who travel across continents and time zones will suffer from jet lag every year. Most people recover after five to seven days. The problem is that until you recover, you may not enjoy your vacation or be effective in your work.

Other factors can worsen the effects of jet lag. If you are under a lot of stress before you leave, you may be worn out before you even get on the plane. If you are anxious about flying it can make jet lag worse.

The severity of jet lag can also depend on what direction you travel and how far you travel. It seems to be easier to adjust to flying west, because you are simply lengthening your day, which demands that you go to bed later and sleep in later. This is pretty easy for most people. When you travel

Most people recover from jet lag after five to seven days.

east, you are behind local time. You are shrinking the day. Traveling east demands that you go to bed earlier and get up earlier, which is more difficult.

The more time zones you traverse, the more difficult the adjustment. If you only travel a single time zone, you will adjust easily. But beyond that, it generally takes about one day to adjust for each time zone you travel east and about one day to adjust for every 1.5 time zones you travel west.

The more time zones you traverse, the more difficult the adjustment.

Coping with Jet Lag

There are three phases to coping with jet lag. The first step involves preparation before you fly, the second involves what you do during the flight, the third covers the steps you take once you arrive.

Before You Fly

First of all, carefully select your flight times. The best thing is to arrive in the late afternoon or early evening. Then you can stay up for a few hours and go to bed at the correct time locally. If you are traveling west, try to arrive in the evening so you can stay up a little later and go to bed at the right time locally. If you are traveling east, try to depart in the evening when you are tired so that you can sleep on the plane and arrive early in the morning. Plan to stay up during the day and do a few low-stress activities. Then go to sleep that night at local time.

Secondly, plan ahead so things don't get too hectic and stressful right before you leave. Make sure you are organized and packed ahead of time. Maintain a good sleep and exercise pattern in the days before you leave. Allow yourself plenty of time to get to the airport. Plan your trip so you don't have any major tasks or decisions facing you on the day you arrive. Give yourself some time to adjust.

Get a clear idea of what time changes you are up against. Graph out the differences between your home time zone and your destination time zone. For example, if you were traveling from New York to Berlin, which is six hours to the east, you could make the following time comparison.

New York	6 A.M.	12 noon	6 P.M.	12 midnight
Berlin	12 noon	6 P.M.	12 midnight	6 A.M.

This chart lets you see clearly how much later your time schedule in Berlin will be and how you need to adjust to this difference.

In the three days before your flight, begin to adjust to the time zone of your destination. If you are flying west, stay up an hour later and wake up an hour later each day. This way, by the time you fly you will have already adjusted to three time zones. If you are flying east, get up an hour earlier and go to bed an hour earlier each day. Also try to shift your meal times an hour each day to coincide with your destination.

If your visit to another time zone is only going to last a day or two, then you may want to forego this process and just stay on your local schedule. If you choose this course of action, then try to plan major events in the new time zone to fit with your home schedule.

Plan ahead to make yourself comfortable while you fly. Wear loose, comfortable clothing suitable for sleep and exercise. Take along neck-support pillows, eyeshades, or earplugs so you can sleep during the flight.

Wear loose, comfortable clothing suitable for sleep and exercise.

While You Are in the Air

When you get on the plane, the first thing to do is to set your watch to the correct time in your destination. This will help you to think about time according to your destination. Drink plenty of water. Cabin air is notoriously dry, and you can easily become dehydrated which puts stress on your body.

Try to get some exercise to keep your muscles loose and your body comfortable. Get up and walk around the plane when it is safe. Do some stretches.

If you are going to sleep, use earplugs and an eye mask. Get a blanket to keep warm and a pillow to support your head. Utilize the many techniques you have learned to help yourself fall asleep. Even if you find it difficult to sleep on the plane, if you do a session of relaxation, you will get some of the rest you need.

If your plan is to stay awake, then you may want to read, converse with a fellow passenger, watch a movie, or do some work. Again, punctuate this activity with some breaks to stretch, walk, and relax.

Avoid drinking alcohol. Alcohol will further dehydrate you and disrupt your sleep. Avoid heavy meals or too many meals. The best thing is to eat at the mealtime for your destination. Avoid caffeine during the flight.

When You Arrive
Make every effort to apply your normal sleep routine to your new environment. Start your day in the morning when the locals do. Eat your meals according to the local schedule. For the first few days, try to eat lighter meals so your digestion can adjust. Plan to go to bed at the right time locally. Resume your normal wind-down, bedtime, and sleep-time routines.

Resume your regular daily exercise cycle. Get out and walk or run or lift weights. Exercise will help you to feel more alert during the day and to sleep better at night.

Use light to help you adjust to your new time zone. If you have traveled east and need to shift back to an earlier

Even if you find it difficult to sleep on the plane, if you do a session of relaxation, you will get some of the rest you need.

wake-up time, then exposure to sunlight in the early morning will reset your sleep clock. Get out in the morning sunlight for at least a half-hour. If there is no sunlight, then use a light box for thirty minutes in the morning.

If you have traveled west and need to stay up later, then exposure to sunlight in the late afternoon will help reset your biological clock. Get out in the late-day sunlight for about thirty minutes, or use a light box for thirty minutes in the late afternoon.

You may also need to do a bit of strategic napping to get you through the first few days. Even a brief nap of twenty to thirty minutes will help you to be more alert and cognitively clear.

If your stay is short and you plan to stay on your home schedule, then you may need to sleep during the day. Be prepared and bring earplugs and eyeshades, or find a hotel that has rooms specifically designed for daytime sleeping with blackout curtains and extra noise control.

When coping with jet lag, consider your sleep personality and learn from your direct experience. Some of the recommendations above may work great for you, while others may not be particularly important or helpful. With experience you will find out the best way to cope with jet lag.

CHILDREN AND OTHER SLEEP CHALLENGES

There are many things that can temporarily impinge on our sleep. Young children can create a sleep challenge as they wake up during the night and get up very early. Parents of young children often sleep with one ear alert to any night-time problems. And when kids are sick, parents may need to listen more carefully and get up more frequently. Fortunately, this is an obligation that most parents take on gladly, and as we noted with shift work, people who are committed to and enjoy their night job cope best with any sleep disruptions.

Taking care of elderly, ill, or handicapped family members or relatives can pose another sleep challenge. And we may encounter work situations when we have to work late and get up early in order to deal with an emergency or meet a deadline.

Keep in mind that sleep is naturally resilient and that a short-term challenge can be dealt with quite easily, particularly if we have good sleep habits. But when the challenge persists, we may need to cope with it in an active and positive manner.

In the case of young children we need to recognize that our sleep is going to be interrupted and shortened for a number of years—not forever, but certainly for a few years. The first step is to simply budget more time for sleep and

> Sleep is naturally resilient. A short-term challenge can be dealt with quite easily, particularly if we have good sleep habits.

In the midst of the demands of caring for children, it will be important to relax your muscles, nervous system, and mind before you drift off to sleep.

cut back on other time-consuming obligations or habits from pre-children days—for example, to forego watching the late news or staying up late reading a book or surfing the Web.

The next step is to maintain a good sleep routine that includes daytime activity and exercise as well as a bedtime routine. You may need to shorten your routine. You may only have ten minutes to do a few stretches or to take a hot bath to wind down. You may only be able to spend a few minutes on your wake-up routine.

In the midst of the demands of caring for children, it will be important to relax your muscles, nervous system, and mind before you drift off to sleep. A few minutes of spiritual reflection and prayer to express thanks for the gift of children can help you to fall asleep with positive emotions. Through prayer, you can surrender your feelings of being overwhelmed and ask for the rejuvenation, strength, and wisdom you need to deal with your current situation.

You will also need to use good sleep techniques to fall back asleep if you are awakened. Be accepting. Talk to yourself in a way to decrease the aggravation. Remind yourself that it is natural to wake up and fall asleep during the night. Relax, rest your mind on something pleasant, and quickly fall back asleep.

A good working relationship with your partner is another key element in overcoming the sleep challenge created by young children. One parent can watch the children while the other exercises or relaxes. Parents can trade off who has to get up at night and who gets up with the early-bird children on the weekends so that the other parent can catch up on her or his sleep.

The strategic use of naps can help to manage a sleep challenge. A brief nap during the midafternoon lull can restore energy. Even a mini-nap of three to five minutes may be helpful. You can sit in a comfortable chair, set a timer for the allotted time, smooth out your breathing, close your eyes, relax your muscles, and ease into whatever kind of sleep comes.

By employing these various strategies, you can continue to get the sleep you need during a sleep challenge. This will help you to maintain your health and vitality. And when you continue to obtain natural, restful sleep, you will be more alert, more productive, and better able to cope with any type of demand during the day.

When you continue to obtain natural, restful sleep, you will be more alert, more productive, and better able to cope with any type of demand during the day.

a daily program for complete, natural sleep

Come let us honor sleep,
that knits up the raveled sleeve of care,
the death of each day's life,
sore labor's bath,
balm of hurt minds,
great nature's second course,
chief nourisher in life's feast.

Congregation of Abraxis

Through the course of this book we have discovered—or perhaps rediscovered—that good sleep is crucially important for our health. During sleep our body rests and repairs itself. When we wake, we feel rejuvenated. Good sleep can boost our powers of concentration, strengthen our problem-solving skills, and enhance our creativity. Good sleep makes us feel more cheerful and optimistic. A restful night of sleep is one of the most simple yet profound pleasures in life.

We have learned that there is an emerging and useful science of sleep. This science has taught us that sleep is an active and organized process that progresses through distinct stages. Sleep is supported by a number of regular daily or circadian rhythms of body temperature and hormone fluctuation regulated by an inner clock in

Good sleep can boost our powers of concentration, strengthen our problem-solving skills, and enhance our creativity.

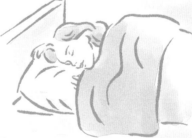

the brain. This inner clock is influenced by the cycles of light and dark. And we have learned that sleep is a resilient, self-correcting process.

We have also learned that we are in the midst of a growing epidemic of sleep deprivation and insomnia. Our environment and culture no longer support good sleep. As a result, we need to actively manage our sleep. We need to start with a vision of what we want to achieve. Our vision should be to get enough sleep, to get quality sleep, and to thoroughly enjoy our sleep. We should be able to fall asleep naturally and sleep straight through the night. We should awake feeling rested and refreshed and feel alert through the day.

Once we have this vision, we are ready to make choices and change our behavior. Let us review the key areas for improving our sleep.

Our vision should be to get enough sleep, to get quality sleep, and to thoroughly enjoy our sleep.

ONGOING SELF-ASSESSMENT

The self-assessment in Chapter 3 is a valuable way to start the process of improving your sleep. But sleep is a dynamic process. From time to time you may want to reevaluate your sleep for a week. Sleep changes as things in your life change. Our sleep may change with the seasons' daylight and temperature changes. Sleep may change if we move or have a new job schedule. And sleep changes as we age.

Because of the responsive nature of sleep, we want to keep an eye on our sleep. This shouldn't become a preoccupation or obsession, but should be a healthy ongoing awareness of how we are sleeping, of what is helping our sleep and what things are harming our sleep.

OPTIMIZING OUR SLEEP ENVIRONMENT

Just as self-assessment is an ongoing process, so is the process of optimizing our sleep environment. We need to continually improve our sleep environment. Perhaps an air conditioner or ceiling fan is wearing out and getting noisy. Perhaps a mattress, sheets, or comforter is aging and needs to be replaced. Our sleep is so important that we not only have to invest in the best furnishings initially, but we need to constantly maintain, replace, and even upgrade our sleep equipment.

We also need to be alert to changes in our environment that can affect our sleep. We may need to add an air conditioner when the weather turns warm or hang blinds in the summer to deal with early morning sunlight. In the winter we may need to add a humidifier to keep the heated air moist.

Just as self-assessment is an ongoing process, so is the process of optimizing our sleep environment.

Your sleep schedule may need to be adjusted to fit your current life situation and demands.

SETTING A SLEEP SCHEDULE

One of the most important steps in improving your sleep is establishing a regular sleep schedule with a designated time for going to bed and a designated time for getting up. This regularity will allow your body clock to synchronize your physiological rhythms to support sleep. This routine will allow you to form habits that will simply make it easier to fall asleep, to sleep well, and to get up easily.

Your sleep schedule may need to be adjusted to fit your current life situation and demands. As your awareness and regulation of your sleep improve, you may be able to fine-tune your schedule so it works even better for you.

Your schedule should always include a wind-down routine, a bedtime routine, a sleep-time routine, a wake-up routine, and a daytime-activity routine. Let us consider the key elements in each of these routines.

The Wind-Down Routine

The purpose of the wind-down routine is to create a transition between the active and alert state of wakefulness and the relaxed, restful state of sleep. Your wind-down routine should begin about thirty to sixty minutes before your bedtime. Remember to eliminate activating behaviors during this time such as surfing the Web or watching violent TV shows.

Express your individuality and create an interesting wind-down routine. Notice what works best, helps you relax, and best prepares you for sleep. You will probably find that some type of stretching or relaxation will be a core element of your wind-down time.

As time goes by, you should begin to look forward to your wind-down time. It should be enjoyable. It should give you the feeling of letting go of the cares of the day, letting go of your revved-up daytime persona, and relaxing and preparing for sleep.

Bedtime Routine

The purpose of your bedtime routine is to establish a chain of behaviors that leads you to sleep. This routine may start with final nighttime actions in your dwelling such as adjusting the thermostat, turning on the dishwasher, and turning out the lights.

Then it is time to get ready for bed. Set up a routine of donning your sleep attire, washing up, brushing your teeth, and performing any final grooming such as brushing your hair. You may want to do a few final stretches or a few minutes of light reading before you turn out the lights. This may be a time for you to read a few lines of scripture or offer an evening prayer.

Your wind-down routine should give you the feeling of letting go of the cares of the day.

Sleep-Time Routine

The purpose of your sleep-time routine is to provide you with a few simple steps that can help you make a natural transition into sleep. Once the lights are out and you are comfortable in your bed, relax your muscles and nervous system. Start with even, smooth diaphragmatic breathing. Do a brief guided relaxation to get rid of any lingering tension in the muscles.

Relax emotionally by simply letting go of negative feelings. Remind yourself that nighttime is not the right time to worry, fret, or even problem-solve. Tune your emotions positively with prayers that express gratitude and ask for protection, strength, and guidance. Let your mind flow through some pleasant sequence that keeps your mind just busy enough so you don't interfere with the natural process of falling asleep.

Wake-Up Routine

The purpose of the wake-up routine is to help you get up at a regular time, to stimulate your daytime alertness, and to reset your biological clock every day. The key element in your wake-up routine is a regular time that should be consistent between your workweek and your weekend.

Before you get out of bed, tune your emotions in a positive direction. Consider the good things you can enjoy during the day. When you get out of bed, face the morning

Relax emotionally by simply letting go of negative feelings.

sunlight, greet the day, and in the process reset your biological clock.

Then you may want to do a few morning stretches, take a brief walk, or exercise. You may want to take a long, enjoyable shower and give yourself plenty of time to get dressed and ready for your day.

You may want to set aside some morning minutes for a period of meditation to clear and balance your mind. Or you may find that the morning is a good time for spiritual study and reflection. You may want to take a few minutes for morning prayers to express your thanks for a new day, to ask for rejuvenation and strength, to seek guidance, wisdom, and protection.

Daytime Activity Routine

Our activity during the day can help or hurt our nighttime sleep. Generally, two things are important. Be active during the day. Try to get some form of exercise. Secondly, get out in the natural light for at least thirty minutes a day.

Activity and exercise during the day are vitally important for good sleep. They help us to feel more alert during the day, setting the stage to feel naturally tired at night. Sleep and activity are the yin and yang of the sleep cycle. They oppose each other, yet complement each other. We want to enjoy both.

Exposure to light is crucial for resetting the biological

Activity and exercise during the day are vitally important for good sleep.

clock. Take a break at work and walk or sit outside for at least ten or fifteen minutes. Get outside for a few minutes in the morning or after work. Even on a cloudy day, the natural light will help.

There are a few things to avoid during the daytime. The first of these is excessive use of caffeine. Try to limit yourself to about two eight-ounce cups of coffee or tea or two sodas per day and don't drink any caffeine after 4 P.M. As a general rule, avoid daytime naps.

THE JOURNEY TOWARD BETTER SLEEP

Improving your sleep is a process. There are three components: *understanding, prioritizing,* and *behavioral choices.* We understand the serious consequences that sleep deprivation can have on our health, safety, vitality, and longevity. We also know that modern life is pushing us down the slippery slope of inadequate and disturbed sleep.

This leads us to the second component. Getting enough sleep and good quality sleep must be absolute priorities in our life. One reason is to help us avoid the health problems and safety risks that poor sleep can bring. The other reason is to feel our very best, to reach our full potential, and to simply enjoy the experience of sleep.

Now is the time to begin the journey toward better sleep. Make some changes. Try some of the approaches.

Getting enough sleep and good quality sleep must be absolute priorities in our life.

Watch the results. Learn more about what works, and keep improving your sleep so you can feel better and have the energy to meet your obligations, reach your goals, and fully enjoy life.

Let us continue this journey with the concluding lines of *Dr. Seuss's Sleep Book*:

> *Ninety-nine zillion*
> *Nine trillion and two*
> *Creatures are sleeping!*
> *So...*
> *How about you?*
>
> *When you put out your light,*
> *Then the number will be*
> *Ninety-nine zillion*
> *Nine trillion and three.*
>
> *Good night.*